QUICK REVIEW IN CLINICAL DENTISTRY

(For AIPG, AIIMS, PGI, BHU and Other State Dental PG Entrance Exams)

QUICK REVIEW IN CLINICAL DENTISTRY

(For AIPG, AIIMS, PGI, BHU and Other State Dental PG Entrance Exams)

Dinamani Khumukcham
Regional Dental College and Hospital
Guwahati

PEEPEE
PUBLISHERS AND DISTRIBUTORS (P) LTD.

Quick Review in Clinical Dentistry

Published by
Pawaninder P. Vij

Peepee Publishers and Distributors (P) Ltd.
Head Office: 160, Shakti Vihar, Pitam Pura, Delhi-110 034 (India)

Corporate Office: 7/31, Ansari Road, Daryaganj
Post Box-7243, New Delhi-110 002 (India)

Ph: 65195868, 23246245, 9811156083

e-mail: peepee160@yahoo.co.in

e-mail: peepee160@rediffmail.com

e-mail: peepee160@gmail.com

www.peepeepub.com

First Edition: **2007**

ISBN: 81-88867-99-3

Printed at
Lordson, C-5/19, Rana Pratap Bagh, Delhi-110 007

To My Father
Khumukcham Haridas Singh
and
My Mother Khumukcham Ibechaobi Devi
for their
Unconditional Love and Support

Preface

Getting a PG seat is a dream for almost all the dental graduates. For this, we need a good study material, proper guidance and a good effort. This book is written in a sincere attempt to provide the dental graduates an up-to-date information and probable questions which can come in the coming exams. All the points in this book should be thoroughly read, revised and remembered. Each point is a question in itself. It covers the maximum and **selected** facts from where the questions are generally made by the question setters. In addition, it contains the past year answers in an easy and memorable way. This book will be highly beneficial for **quick revision** and **clearing concepts** of the dental subjects.

As the saying goes:

"Awake, arise and rest not till your goal is reached." So dear friends, "Let us hope for the best and prepare for the worst."

My best wishes to all those who are preparing for PG entrance exams and hope this book will help you in converting your dream into a reality.

Dinamani Kh.

e-mail : dk_noi@yahoo.co.in

Acknowledgements

My heartfelt thanks goes to the God, our saviour for enabling me to complete this book in time.

I give my sincere thanks to my family members for their untiring support, love and belief on me.

I am thankful to Dr. P.D. Bora, Prinicipal, the Regional Dental College and Hospital, Guwahati for his encouragement during my college days. I thank all my teachers for their valuable guidance.

My sincere thanks goes to Dr. Navin Kumar Choudhury, the Bapuji Dental College and Hospital, Davangere (author of AIIMS DENTAL MAY-2006 and PGI-DENTAL JUNE-2006) for his advice and encouragement in writing this book.

I am very much thankful to my seniors Dr. L. Hector, Dr. Robinson, Dr. Shamananda, Dr. Anitarani, Dr. Apwong Golmei, Dr. James, Dr. Nilmani for their guidance and help.

Words fail to express my feelings when I thank my batchmates Dr. Herojit, Dr. Surajit, Dr. Lalrammawia, Dr. Tage, Dr. Kaling, Dr. Heibor, Dr. Seto, Dr. Bency, Dr. Jaba, Dr. Epsita, Dr. Shivanjali, Dr. Zaii, Dr. Mahlui, Dr. Easter, Dr. Mezhuno, Dr. Til and Dr. Viphre for their support and co-operation during my college days.

I also give my heartfelt thanks to Dr. Sumit Lavaria, Kasturba Medical College, Manipal.

I am sincerely thankful to Dr. Birendra Kumar and Dr. Ashish Kumar, Patna Dental College and Hospital, Patna.

I have no words to express my gratitude to Dr. Chirag Desai, M.P. Shah Medical College, Jamnagar for his inspiration.

I show my gratitude to Dr. Varun Gupta, J.N. Medical College, Aligarh for his kind help in bringing out this book.

I am deeply indebted to my brothers Kh. Priyokumar (Boge), Priyojit, my sister Bhanumati, my sister-in-laws Pratima and Nandini. I am very thankful to the God for giving me a brother like Priyokumar, for his guidance and encouragement throughout my career. Life would have been more difficult without him.

I also give my heartfelt thanks to my uncle Padmashree L. Nabakishore (Chief Physician, Urinary Tract and Stone Case Centre) for his encouragement and support.

Lastly, I give my sincere thanks to the publishers Mr. Pawaninder Pal Vij, Director, Peepee Publishers and Distributors (P) Ltd., New Delhi and all staff members who are involved in bringing out this book.

Contents

Suggested Readings

1.	Oral Surgery	-	Neelima Anil Malik Peterson
2.	Local Anesthesia	-	Malamed, Monheim
3.	Oral Radiology	-	White & Pharoah
4.	Fractures of Mandible and Maxilla	-	Killey (Peter Banks)
5.	Endodontics	-	Grossman, Ingle, Cohens
6.	Orthodontics	-	Profitt, Bhalajhi, Rani
7.	Pediatric Dentistry	-	Sobha Tandon, McDonald, Damle
8.	Complete Denture	-	Boucher, Winkler
9.	Removable Partial Denture	-	McCracken, Stewart
10.	Fixed Partial Denture	-	Rosenstiel, Tylman
11.	Periodontics	-	Carranza
12.	Community Dentistry	-	Soben Peter
13.	PSM	-	Park & Park
14.	Conservative Dentistry	-	Sturdevant, Sikri

CHAPTER ONE

Oral Surgery

(Including Oral Radiology, LA, Fractures)

- Completed tomography was first described by Johann Radon.
- The principle of diagnostic imaging is As Low As Reasonably Achievable or ALARA for X-exposure.
- Purcell and Block described magnetic resonance imaging (MRI).
- MRI is non-ionizing radiation.
- Sagittal plane is the standard plane of MRI used to study TMT disc deformities.
- In Scintigraphy, radionuclide ^{99m}Technetium **labelled** phosphate or ^{67}Gallium is used.
- **CT scan** is considered the **gold** standard of diagnostic imaging.
- The most commonly used blade in oral surgery is No. 15 blade while No. 3 Bard Parker Blade handle is the most commonly used blade handle.
- The basic purpose of a suture is to hold severed tissues in close approximation until the healing process provides the wound with sufficient strength to withstand stress.

- Isopropyl alcohol is used to preserve gut because it is highly susceptible to enzymatic degradation.
- Gut suture is absorbed by proteolytic degradation and phagocytosis while polyglycolic acid and polyglactin 910 are resorbed by hydrolysis.
- Chromic gut as compared to plain gut has slightly increased strength, prolonged rate of absorption, and lesser stimulation of tissue reaction.
- Braided **polyglycolic** acid and polyglactin 910 are the strongest of the absorbable materials.
- Silk undergoes slow **proteolysis** when implanted and is the most popular suture material for intraoral use or mucosal sutures.
- **Nylon** is the most popular skin suture material.
- The initial body response to sutures is identical in the first 4 to 7 days, regardless of the suture material.
- The most commonly used suture method is the interrupted suture.
- The figure of 8 suture is used over extraction sites for protection of the surgical area and adaptation of the gingival papillae around the adjacent teeth.
- In subcuticular suture, an absorbable 4-0 suture material is used.
- Removal of skin sutures are done after 7 to 10 days while mucosal sutures are removed after 5 to 7 days.
- The test organism used for checking the efficiency of autoclave (moist heat sterilization) is Bacillus steorothermophilus. ***(BHU '06)***
- Hand **scrub** is the first step towards **aseptic** technique.
- Ethylene oxide destroys organisms by alkylation.

- 70% alcohol as disinfectant is more effective than higher concentrations, because the presence of water speeds the protein denaturation.
- Differences in the technique of electrodesiccation, electrocoagulation, electrosurgery and electrocautery.

Electrodesiccation (electrofulguration)	*Electro-coagulation*	*Electro-surgery*	*Electro-cautery*
High frequency alternating current (A.C.) of high voltage and low amperage is used	High frequency damped A.C. with low amperage and voltage than that of electro-desiccation is used	High frequency A.C. undamped or rectified is used	Low voltage and low amperage is used

- Benzalkonium chloride is the most commonly used antiseptic.

TEMPOROMANDIBULAR JOINT

- Development of the temporomandibular joint starts at approximately 10-12 weeks.
- The articulating surfaces of the condylar processes and fossae are covered with avascular fibrous cartilage.
- Avascular articular disc divides the articular space into lower compartment and upper compartment.
- Non-articular surfaces of the temporomandibular joint are covered with periosteum.
- The volume of lower joint space is about 0.9 ml while volume of upper joint space is about 1.2 ml.
- Non-articular surfaces of the temporomandibular joint are covered with periosteum.
- Blood supply of temporamandibular joint is branches from superficial temporal and maxillary arteries.

- Nerve supply of temporomandibular joint is auriculotemporal nerve, masseteric nerve and a branch from posterior deep temporal nerve.
- Ehlers-Danlos syndrome is a rare inherited disorder of the connective tissue, in which recurrent dislocation of the **TMJ** is seen.
- Surgical techniques for treatment of TMJ ankylosis are:
  1. **Condylectomy:** It is advocated in cases of fibrous ankylosis
  2. **Gap arthroplasty:** A gap of 1 cm is created by sectioning the bone upto the level of previous joint space.
  3. **Interpositional arthroplasty:** A barrier of autogenous or alloplastic is inserted in the gap created to reduce the risk of recurrence and to maintain the vertical height of the ramus.
- **TMJ arthroscopy** was made popular by **Ohnishi**.

CYST AND TUMOURS OF JAWS AND ORAL TISSUES

- Robinson popularized the term primordial cyst and Phillipsen coined keratocyst.
- Total protein of odontogenic keratocyst is less than **4 gm/100 ml.**
- Paget coined the term dentigerous cyst.
- Weathers and Waldron recognised the botryoid odontogenic cyst.
- Gorlin first described the calcifying epithelial odontogenic cyst.

- Thoma first described globulomaxillary cyst.
- Taffe and Lichetenstein first described aneurysmal bone cyst.
- Nasolabial cyst is a soft tissue cyst. So, it does not exhibit any radiographic change.
- Radiograph of globulomaxillary cyst reveals an inverted, pear-shaped radiolucent area between the roots of the upper lateral incisor and canine.
- Heart-shaped or small round radiolucent area between the roots of the upper central incisors is the radiographic appearance of nasopalatine duct cyst.
- Aneurysmal bone cyst shows a typical "honeycomb appearance" on radiograph.
- Lateral periodontal cyst shows teardrop-shaped radiolucent area on radiograph.
- Dentigerous cyst sometimes transform into amelo-blastoma.
- Radicular cyst develops from the epithelial cell rests of Malassez.
- **Focal epithelial hyperplasia** is also called **Heck's disease.**
- Three variants of non lipid reticuloendothelioses are:
  1. Eosinophilic granuloma (histiocytosis X localized to bone).
  2. Hand-Schuller-Christian disease (chronic disseminated histiocytosis X).
  3. Letterer-Siwe disease (acute disseminated histiocytosis X).
- Brown tumour of hyperparathyroidism is so called because of the presence of hemosiderin.

- Extensive 'punched-out' areas of destruction or map like geographic involvement of the skull is present in Hand-Schuller-Christian disease.
- The triad of Hand-Schuller-Christian disease are exophthalmos, bone lesions, and diabetes insipidus.
- **"Floating tooth" phenomenon** due to complete alveolar bone loss is found in **eosinophilic granuloma**.
- Verocay bodies present in neurilemoma are steplike or whorled formations of nuclei surrounding acellular hyalinized collagen masses.
- Antoni A and Antoni B pattern of Schwann cells are present in neurilemoma.
- Neurilemoma is most commonly occurred on the posterior body and ramus of the mandible.
- Radiotherapy is contraindicated in the treatment of cherubism due to possibility of sarcoma formation and interference with growth in children.
- Cherubism was first described by Jones.
- **Cuzack** first recognized **ameloblastoma**.
- Churchill and Ivy coined the term 'ameloblastoma'.
- Most common sites for spread of ameloblastoma are lungs and it is due to aspiration of tumour cells during extensive manipulation.
- Liesegang rings are present in calcifying epithelial odontogenic tumour (Pindborg tumour).

LOCAL ANAESTHESIA

- **Melzack** and **Wall** proposed the gate control theory of pain.

- The injected local anaesthetic drug must come into contact with at least 8 to 10 mm of the nerve for maximum effect.
- The specific receptor theory is the most popular theory for the mechanism of action of local anesthetics.
- The local anesthetics produce a loss of function in the following order: **pa**in, **t**emperature, **to**uch, **pro**prioception, and **s**keletal muscle tone. (Mnemonic: **PaT**-To-**ProS**).
- All the local anesthetic agents have vasodilator properties except cocaine which is vasoconstriction in action.
- Ester group of local anesthetics undergoes hydrolysis in the plasma and is catalyzed by the enzyme plasma cholinesterase.
- Amide type of local anesthetics undergoes biotransformation in the liver by microsomal enzymes.
- Lidocaine is synthesized by Lofgren and its melting point is 69°C. It is combined with hydrochloride salt to make it water soluble readily.
- The major urinary metabolic of lidocaine is 4-hydroxy-2, 6-dimethylaniline.
- Chemical name of lidocaine is **diethyl**-2, 6-**dimethyl-acetanilid**.
- Procaine is incompatible with sulfonamides because PABA is a metabolite of procaine and sulfonamides acts by competitive antagonism with PABA.
- 2-chloroprocaine is recommended for use in children because of its shorter duration of anesthesia.
- Prilocaine is contraindicated in patients with congenital or idiopathic methemoglobinemia because

orthotuluidine, a metabolite of prilocaine produce methemoglobin.

- Long acting anesthetics like bupivacaine, etidocaine etc. are contraindicated in children because of danger of traumatizing soft tissue by biting, chewing, and so forth.

Water insoluble topical anesthetics	*Water soluble topical anesthetics*
1. Benzocaine	1. Benzyl alcohol
2. Lidocaine base	2. Tetracaine Hel (Pontocaine)
	3. Lidocaine HCl

- The vasoconstrictors used in dental local anesthetic solutions are:
  1. Pyrocatechin derivatives—epinephrine and norepinephrine.
  2. Benzol derivatives—levonordefrin (Neo-cobefrin).
  3. Phenol derivatives—phenylephrine (Neo-synephrine).
- Grading system of patient's physical status adopted by the American Society of Anesthesiologists:

PS I : A normal healthy patient.

PS II : A patient with mild systemic disease.

PS III : A patient with severe systemic disease that limits activity but is not incapacitating.

PS IV : A patient with an incapacitating systemic disease that is a constant threat to life.

PS V : A moribund patient not expected to survive 24 hours with or without operation.

E : Patients treated on emergency, the letter E follows the physical status designation.

- The absolute contraindication of local anesthetic solution containing a vasoconstrictor is patient with untreated hyperthyroidism. These patients are highly sensitive to sympathomimetic agents and a thyroid storm may occur.

EXTRACTION OF TEETH

- Preoperative radiograph is advised in patients with cleido-cranical dysostosis because pseudo-anodontia and hooked roots occur in this condition.
- The most important contraindication to local anesthesia is the presence of acute infection at the site of operation.
- During extraction of maxillary tooth, the dental chair should be adjusted so that the site of operation is about 3 inches below the shoulder level of the operator while during extraction of mandibular tooth, it should be about 6 inches below the level of the operator's elbow.
- **The most widely** used instruments for extraction of teeth are the **dental forceps.**
- The blades of upper premolar forceps are mirror-images of each other and the same instrument can be used to extract both right and left maxillary premolars.
- Primary rotatory movement is done to loosen maxillary central incisor and mandibular second premolar from socket. If it resist rotation, buccolingual movement is done to avoid spiral fracture of the tooth-root.
- If the patient's mouth is opened too widely while trying to extract maxillary third molar, the coronoid process may interfere with access and increase the difficulty. So the patient is asked to half closes the mouth and deviates his mandible towards the side of extraction

so that coronoid process moves away from the site of operation.

- Elevators are used on the lever and fulcrum principle.
- Rongeur forceps are used as bone scissors.
- Sutures used to repair an oro-antral communication are left in situ for at least 10 days unless they become infected.
- Hilton's method of draining an abscess ensures that no blood-vessel or nerve is damaged.
- Composition of Whitehead's varnish (Pigmentum Iodoform Compositum).
  1. Benzoin – 3g
  2. Prepared storax – 2 g
  3. Balsam of Tolu – 1.5 g
  4. Iodoform – 3 g
  5. Solvent Ether – 28.4 ml
- The **most common cause** for extraction of teeth is **caries** and next is periodontal disease.
- Roots of the second and third molar may be displaced in the submandibular space through a perforation in the lingual surface of the mandible.
- Dry socket (alveolarosteitis) generally starts on the third to fifth day after extraction of the tooth and, if untreated, will last for 7 to 14 days.
- The best time to remove impacted third molar teeth is when radiograph shows the roots of the third molars to be half to two thirds formed i.e. 16 and 17 years of age.
- **Fry** developed **lingual split-bone technique** for removal of deeply positioned horizontal and disto-angular mandibular third molar impactions.

- Miller elevators and Potts elevators are used for removal of impacted and unerupted maxillary third molars.
- The most common location of **developmentally** displaced mandibular third molars is in the ascending ramus.
- Mandibular and maxillary third molars sometimes develop at a distance from their normal location because of unusual proliferation of the odontogenic epithelium before development of the tooth germ.
- Tumours that develop from dental follicle are odontoma and ameloblastoma.
- Bolk coined the term mesiodens (mesiodentes).
- Difficulty Index for removal of impacted lower third molars.

Classification	*Difficulty index value*
a. Angulation	
Mesioangular	1
Horizontal	2
Vertical	3
Distoangular	4
b. Depth	
A	1
B	2
C	3
c. Space available	
Class I	1
Class II	2
Class III	3

- Difficulty Index
  1. Very difficult : 7 to 10 (total value)
  2. Moderately difficulty : 5 to 7
  3. Minimally difficulty : 3 to 4

- In winter's WAR lines:
  1. **White line** represents the line joining the buccal cusps of erupted molars and going posterior over third molar region.
  2. **Amber line** represents the bone level covering the impacted tooth. The line runs at the level of the crest of the interdental septum between the molars and extended posteriorly distal to third molar.
  3. **Red line** is the line drawn perpendicular from amber line to an imaginary point, where elevator will be applied.

  Extraction of the impacted tooth is difficult if the length of the red line is more than 5 mm. Addition of 1 mm i.e. 6 mm renders the removal of the tooth three times more difficult.

FRACTURES OF THE MANDIBLE

- The **most common** site for mandibular fracture is **the neck of the condyle.**
- Guardsman fracture is the most common multiple fracture of mandible. It is caused by a fall on the mid-point of the chin resulting in fractures of the symphysis and both condyles. These fractures are commonly seen in epileptics, elderly patients and sometimes in soldiers who faint on parade.
- Sudden refles contracture of the temporalis muscle can cause fracture of the coronoid process.
- A frontal impact force of 425 lb on the mandible produces fracture of the condylar neck.
- The most important structure in determining the stability or unstability of a mandibular fracture is the periosteum.

- Lateral pterygoid muscle causes displacement of condylar head medially and forward when the condylar neck fracture occurs.
- The extreme downward and backward angulation of the anterior part of the mandible under the influence of the digastric and the mylohyoid muscles is called '**bucket handle**' displacement. It is peculiar to the thin edentulous mandible of elderly patient.
- The periosteal blood supply to the mandible becomes increasingly important with ageing as the inferior dental artery slowly diminishes in size.
- Facial palsy of the lower motor neurone type results when facial nerve is damaged by direct trauma over the mandibular ramus.
- Swelling and ecchymosis indicate the site of any mandibular fracture.
- **Primary bone healing** takes place when immobilization is done with **compression plates.**
- Dental wiring is used for immobilization of fracture of mandible when the patient has a complete or almost complete set of suitably shaped teeth. Stretching of the wire about 10% is required to prevent slack after being in position a few days.
- Arch bars are used when there is insufficient number of suitably shaped teeth.
- Winter, Jelenko and Erich type bars are prefabricated arch bars.
- The Brenthurst splint is an example of bone clamps.
- Cap splints are indicated in:
  1. Fracture of mandible in patients with extensive and advanced periodontal disease.

2. Fractures of the tooth-bearing segment and bilateral displaced fractures of the condylar neck.
3. Missing of a portion of the body of the mandible with substantial soft-tissue loss.

- Circumferential wires are used to immobilize oblique fractures of the endentulous mandible.
- In children before puberty, the treatment of mandibular fractures is generally of a conservative nature.
- On radiograph non-union of fracture is seen as eburnation i.e. rounding off and sclerosis of the bone ends.
- The miniplates used for immobilization of mandibular fractures have a thickness of 0.9 mm with holes of minimum diameter 2.1.

FRACTURES OF THE MIDDLE THIRD OF THE FACIAL SKELETON

- A force of 140 lb can cause fracture of the maxilla.
- If the middle third of the facial skeleton is removed, the frontal bone and body of the sphenoid form an inclined plane which lies at an angle of about 45° to the occlusal plane.
- Hooding of the eye occurs in zygomatic and Le Fort III fractures.
- **Epiphora** occurs in Le Fort II, Le Fort III and nasal complex fractures.
- The most important factor controlling the patency of the airway in a patient with facial injuries is the level of consciousness.

- **Teasdale** and **Jennett** described **'Glasgow coma scale'**.
- Repair of soft-tissue lacerations associated with fractures of the maxilla should be done within 1-7 hours of injury before oedema has occurred.
- Indications for tracheostomy in maxillofacial injuries:
  1. Necessity of prolonged artificial ventilation.
  2. Facilitation of anaesthesia for surgical repair in major injuries.
  3. Obstruction of the airway from laryngeal oedema.
  4. Extensive haemorrhage into the airway.
- Retrograde amnesia and anterograde amnesia are **indicative** of cerebral damage.
- A tramline pattern on the face and a halo effect on the pillow and sheets is produced by leaking of blood and cerebrospinal fluid from the nose.
- Persistent leak of cerebrospinal fluid can be detected by intrathecal administration of radioactive isotope $99m_{Tc}$.
- Circumorbital ecchymosis occurs in zygomatic fracture, Le Fort II and Le Fort III fractures.
- Hess chart records the degree of diplopia.
- **Water's projection** of the face shows **'hanging drop' sign** in cases of orbital floor fracture. The opacity that appears on the radiograph is made up of extravasated blood and herniated fat.
- Bilateral subconjunctival ecchymosis is associated with Le Fort II, Le Fort III, naso-ethmoidal complex fractures. ***(AIPG '06)***
- Bilateral circumorbital ecchymosis occurs in nasal complex fracture, Le Fort I and Le Fort II fractures.

- '**Cracked-pot**' sound on percussion of the upper teeth occurs in Le Fort I, Le Fort II and Le Fort III fractures.
- '**Moon-face**' appearance is seen in Le Fort II and Le Fort III fractures.
- Le Fort I fracture is also called Guerin fracture while Pyramidal fracture is the another name of Le Fort II fracture.
- Gillies temporal approach is used for reduction of recent fracture of zygomatic complex. The instrument used is Bristow's elevator.
- Transosseous wiring at the infra-orbital rim is usually done with 0.35 mm soft stainless-steel wire.
- Orbital blow-out fracture was described by Smith and Regan.
- Orbital blow-in fracture was described by Dingman and Natvig.
- Enophthalmos greater than 3 mm requires surgical intervention.
- Walsham and Asche's forceps are used for reduction of nasal complex fracture.
- Plaster of Paris splint and lead plates are used for fixation of nasal complex fractures.
- Rowe's disimpaction forceps are used for reduction of Le Fort I and sometimes Le Fort II and Le Fort III fractures.
- Halo-frames is devised by Crawford.
- Impacted Le Fort I fracture is also called telescopic fracture. It is cause by a force transmitted via a blow to the lower jaw.

ORAL RADIOLOGY

- X-rays, gamma rays, ultraviolet rays, visible light, infrared radiation, microwaves and radiowaves are all examples of electromagnetic radiation.
- The sharpness of the radiographic image increases, as the size of the radiation source–the focal spot–decreases.
- The speed of the electrons increases as the Kilovoltage peak (KvP) increases. So greater penetrability of the X-ray beam through matter is observed.
- Bremsstrahlung radiations are produced by the sudden stopping or slowing of high-speed electrons at the target. It is the primary source of X-ray photons from an X-ray tube.
- The quantity of radiation produced by an X-ray tube is directly proportional to the tube current (mA).
- The half value layer (HVL) is the thickness of an absorber required to reduce by one half the number of X-ray photons passing through it.
- Quality of an X-ray refers to the mean energy of an X-ray beam.
- The aluminium filter is used to remove lower-energy photons from X-ray beam (1.5 mm thick aluminium for 70 KVp and 2.5 mm of aluminium for higher voltages).
- A lead collimator is used to reduce the size of the X-ray beam and therefore the patient exposure.
- Collimation improves image quality by reducing **compton scattering**.

- Units of measurement:

Quality	*SI units*
1. Exposure	Coulomb per kilogram
2. Absorbed dose	Gray
3. Equivalent dose/Effective dose	Sievert
4. Radioactivity	Becquerel

- Exposure is the capacity of radiation to ionize air.
- Equivalent dose is used to compare the biologic effects of different types of radiation on a tissue or organ.
- Effective dose is used to estimate the risk in humans.
- Hydroperoxyl free radicals and hydrogen peroxide are considered to be major toxins produced in the tissues by ionizing radiations.
- Early precursor cells of erythroblastic series and basal cells of the oral mucous membrane are the most radiosensitive.
- Neurons, striated muscle cells, mature erythrocyte and optic lens are radioresistant i.e. low radiosensitive.
- **Salivary flow reduces to zero** at a radiation dose of **60 Gy (6000 rads).** ***(AIPG'05)***
- Radiations therapy to oral region leads to increase in streptococcus mutans, Lactobacillus, and candida.
- For reducing radiation caries, topical 1% neutral sodium fluoride gel in custom made tray is applied on the teeth for 5 minutes daily.
- About 44% of buffering capacity of saliva falls during radiations therapy.
- Cardiovascular and central nervous system symptoms starts to appear at a radiation dose of 50 Gy.

- The most radiosensitive period for inducing developmental abnormalities is between 18 and 45 days of gestation i.e. during the period of organogenesis.
- **Human brain** is most sensitive at **8 to 15 weeks** postconception.
- Image contrast increases when kilovoltage is decreased.
- Radiographs are best viewed in a semidarkened room with light transmitted only through the films.
- X-ray film has two principal components: emulsion and base. The emulsion is sensitive to X-rays, visible light and records the radiographic image. The base is a plastic supporting material onto which the emulsion is coated.
- The thickness of base of ultraspeed film is 0.18 mm and is made of polyester polyethylene terephthalate.
- Bitewing radiograph is useful for detecting interproximal caries and evaluating the height of alveolar bone.
- Radiographic density is the overall degree of darkening of an exposed film.
- Radiographic contrast is the difference in densities between light and dark regions on a radiograph.
- **Radiographic noise** is the appearance of uneven density of a uniformly exposed radiographic film.
- Sharpness is the ability of a radiograph to define an edge precisely while resolution is the ability of a radiograph to record separate structures that are close together.

- Composition of developing solution:

1. Developer	Hydroquinone or phenidone
2. Activator	Sodium or potassium hydroxide
3. Preservative	Sodium sulfite
4. Restrainer (antifog agent)	Potassium or sodium bromide

- Composition of fixing solution:

1. Clearing agent	Ammonium thiosulfate
2. Acidifier	Acetic acid
3. Preservative	Sodium or ammonium sulfite
4. Hardener	Aluminium salts

- The processing tank of X-ray film should be maintained at temperature between 60° and 75°F.
- **Godfrey Hounsfield** invented computerized axial transverse scanning (CAT scan).
- The lamina dura is wider and more dense around the roots of teeth in heavy occlusion, and thinner and less dense around teeth not subjected to **occlusal** function.
- Stereoscopy was introduced by Mackenzie Davidson in 1898 but stereoscopic technique in dental radiography was first described by Ivy in 1917. Its uses are:
  1. Determination of root configuration of teeth.
  2. Evaluation of bony pocket.
  3. Assessment of relationship of mandibular canal to the roots of unerupted third molars.
  4. Assessment of bone shape for implant placement.
- Foreshotening of radiographic image results when the central ray is perpendicular to the film but the object is not parallel with the film.

- Elongation of a radiographic image results when the central ray is perpendicular to the object but not the film.

Extraoral skill projection	*Main structure seen*
1. Lateral projection	Calvarium and base of the skull, shape and depth of Sella Turcica, soft tissues of nasopharynx
2. Waters projection (occipitomental projection)	Maxillary, frontal and ethmoidal sinuses. If taken with mouth open, sphenoidal sinus is also seen
3. Reverse Towne's projection	Neck of condyle
4. Submentovertex	Base of skull, position and orientation of condyle, **sphenoidal sinus**, lateral wall of maxillary sinus, zygomatic arc
5. Oblique lateral projections	Mandibular body and mandibular ramus

- **TMJ** arthrography is indicated for gaining information about articular disk position, function, morphology and the integrity of diskal attachments. It is contraindicated in patients allergic to **nonionic** iodine contrast agent.
- Bony ankylosis, developmental abnormalities and joint space calcifications of temporomandibular joint are best detected with computed tomography (CT scan).
- Projections of TMJ and their use:

Transcranial	*Transpharyngeal*	*Transorbital*
Provides sagittal view of lateral aspects of condyle and temporal component	Provides sagittal view of medial pole of the condyle	Provides an anterior view of the TMJ

Systemic disease	*Radiographic appearance*
1. Hyperparathyroidism	Ground glass appearances due to numerous, small, randomly oriented trabecular. ***(AIPG '06)*** Loss of lamina dura
2. Sickle cell anemia	Thinning of cancellous trabeculae and cortical bone; widening of the diploic space in the skull; osteoporosis of jaws. Hair-on-appearance (5% of cases)
3. Thalassemia	Generalized granular appearance of skull and thickening of diploic space, Hair-on-end appearance
4. Hypophosphatemia (renal tubular disorders resulting in excessive loss phosphorus)	Large pulp chambers and root canals; periapical and periodontal abscesses occur frequently
5. Hypophosphatasia (reduced production or defective function of alkaline phosphatase)	Large pulp chambers and root canal; Gyral or convolutional markings that resemble hammered copper and appear as multiple radiolucent areas of the calvarium. Brachycephalic shape of skull
6. Hyperthyroidism	Early eruption of teeth premature loss of primary teeth
7. Hypothyroidism	Delayed eruption of teeth, periodontal disease, loss of teeth, enlarged tongue
8. Hypoparathyroidism	Delayed eruption of teeth, calcification of basal ganglia

- Mucoepidermoid carcinoma is the most common malignant salivary gland tumor (35%) Cavitary sialectasia and ductal displacement may be noted on sialographic images.
- Pleomorphic adenomas account for 75% of salivary gland tumors. Of these, 80% are found in the parotid gland, 4% in submandibular gland, 1% in sublingual gland, and 10% in the minor salivary gland.
- **Hemangioma** is the most frequently occurring nonepithelial salivary neoplasm. **Phleboliths** are common in this tumor.
- Sialography is indicated for the evaluation of chronic inflammatory diseases and ductal pathoses. It is

contraindicated in acute infection and known sensitivity to iodine containing compounds.

- Accentuation of antegonial notch and steep mandibular angle is seen in mandibulofacial dysostosis or Treacher collins syndrome.
- In Craniofacial dysostosis or Crouzon's disease, the maxilla is underdeveloped, resulting in crowding of dentition. Increased intracranial pressure from the brain due to absence of sutures leads to prominent **cranial markings** of the inner surface of the cranial vault. It appears as multiple radiolucent depressions which results in beaten metal appearance.
- Osteoma cutis is a rare soft tissue ossification in the skin. Face is the most common site while tongue is the most common intraoral site.
- Fibrous dysplasia is most commonly located on the posterior maxilla. It appears as "ground glass" on extraoral radiographs and as "orange peel" on intraoral views.
- "Sharpened pencil appearance" of the condyle is seen on the radiograph of rheumatoid arthritis. It is due to erosion of the anterior and posterior condylar surfaces at the attachment of the synovial lining.
- 'Ely cysts' are small, round, radiolucent areas with irregular margins surrounded by a varying of increased density, deep to the articulating surfaces of the condyle seen on the radiograph of **osteoarthritis**. They are not true cysts but they are areas of degeneration that contain fibrous tissue, granulation tissue, and osteoid.
- Osteophytes are bony proliferation that occurs at the periphery of the articulating surface of the condyle in the later course of osteoarthritis.

- Articular disk perforation is detected with the help of arthrography.
- Internal derangement of the articular disk is seen with the help of Magnetic Resonance Imaging (MRI) or arthrography.
- "**Toadstool appearance**" with marked flattening and apparent elongation of the articulating condylar surface and posterior inclination of the condyle and neck is seen on the radiograph of Boering's arthrosis or Juvenile arthrosis.
- External root resorption is present on the radiographic pictures of hypoparathyroidism and hypothyroidism.
- Delayed eruption of teeth is found in:
  1. **O**steopetrosis (marble bone disease).
  2. **Hypo**thyroidism.
  3. **Hypo**parathyroidism.
  4. **R**ickets.

  Mnemonic: **HypRO**
- Hypocalcification and hypoplasia of teeth are present in the following systemic diseases:
  1. Rickets.
  2. Hypophosphatasia.
  3. Hypophosphatemia.
  4. Renal Osteodystrophy.
- Loss of teeth is a distinct feature of in:
  1. Hypothyroidism.
  2. Hyperthyroidism.
  3. Hypophosphatemia.
  4. Renal Osteodystrophy.
  5. Hypophosphatasia.

- Punched out lesions on radiograph are present in multiple myeloma and sometimes in eosinophic granuloma.
- Cementoblastoma are mixed radiolucent—radiopaque lesions that may have a **wheel spoke** pattern on radiograph.
- Odontogenic myxoma is often associated with unerupted or congenitally missing tooth.
- Radiation doses above **50 Gy** are usually required to cause **osteoradionecrosis**.
- The first radiographic evidence of acute osteomyelitis is a slight decrease in the density of the involved bone with a loss of sharpness of the existing trabeculae.
- The radiographic appearance of radiation caries is dark radiolucent shadows appearing at the necks of teeth, most obvious on the mesial and distal aspects.
- Calcium hydroxide preparations without barium, lead or zinc appear radiolucent and resemble caries. ***(AIPG '06)***
- Relative patient exposure of bitewing radiograph is 10 times that of intraoral periapical radiograph.
- For full mouth radiographic examination of a pregnant lady, the fetal exposure is about 1 mGy provided the lady is shielded with a leaded apron.
- **Cervical burnout** caused by overexposure or decreased X-ray absorption appear to be carious on radiograph. It is diffuse radiolucent areas with ill-defined borders on the mesial or distal aspect of teeth between the enamel and alveolar crest.

ADDITIONAL HIGH YIELD FACTS

- Epicenter of the bone destruction in Langerhan's cell Histiocytosis is in the midroot region of tooth resulting in "**ice cream scoop**" appearance.
- **Sialography** was first described and performed by Carpy.
- Frey's syndrome is a condition in which there is flushing and sweating of the skin in the area distributed by auriculotemporal nerve. It has no treatment.
- In Pierre Robin Syndrome, triad of cleft palate, mandibular micrognathia and glossoptosis is present.
- The shape of maxillary sinus at birth is tubular and at adult is pyramidal.
- Maxillary sinus reaches its normal adult size by 15 years. It is lined by pseudostratified ciliated columnar epithelium (Schneiderian membrane).
- Symptoms of fresh oroantral communication:
  a. Escape of fluids from mouth to nose on the site of extraction.
  b. Epistaxis.
  c. Escape of air.
  d. Change in the voice.
  e. Severe pain.
- Treatment of oroantral communication and oroantal fistula of long duration more than 4 weeks is surgical closure. ***(BHU'06)***
- **Danger space** is potential space between the alar and prevertebral fascia. Oropharyngeal infections can spread from retropharyngeal space to posterior mediastinum through danger space.

- **The space of burns (suprasternal space)** is the potential space between two layers of superficial fascia that are attached to the clavicle. The two layers of superficial fascia are attached to the anterior and posterior border of the manubrium sterni.
- **Fothergill's disease** is trigeminal neuralgia.
- **Neuropraxia**—There is no axonal degeneration distal to the area of injury; paresthesia is present. ***(PGI '06)***
- **Axonotmesis**—There is loss of continuity of some axons, which undergo Wallerian degeneration distal to the site of injury; hypoesthesia and dysaesthesias develop in the area supplied by the nerve.
- **Neurotmesis**—There is Wallerian degeneration of all axons distal to the injury; paralysis and anaesthesia of all nerve impulses develop.

Type of orthognathic surgery	*Indications*
1. Mandibular body osteotomy (both posterior and anterior)	Correction of Class III malocclusion (Mandibular setback)
2. Subcondylar vertical osteotomy	Mandibular setback
3. Intraoral vertical ramus osteotomy (IVRO) and Inverted L osteotomy	Mandibular setback ***(PGI '06)***
4. Intraoral Modified Sagittal split osteotomy	Both setback or advancement of mandible
5. Le Fort I osteotomy	Repositioning of entire dentoalveolar segment of the maxilla superiorly, inferiorly, anteriorly and posteriorly, while at the same time segmentalizing it to widen, narrow, level or improve arch symmetry

- **Horshoe-shaped osteotonus** is a modification of Le Fort I osteotomy in which superior positioning of the maxilla is done by leaving the nasal floor intact.
- **Behrman's bump** is a bony prominence corresponding to the side of lingual and mandibular foramen on the lateral surface of the mandibular ramus.

Osteotomy procedure	*Person who described or performed it*
1. Anterior mandibular osteotomy	S.P. Hullihen
2. Subcondylar vertical osteotomy	Caldwell-Letterman
3. Intraoral vertical Ramus osteotomy and Inverted L osteotomy	Winstanley
4. Sagittal Split Osteotomy	Trauner and Obwegeser
5. Anterior maxillary osteotomy	Cohn Stock

- Nitrous oxide was first prepared by Priestley and it is the only inorganic gas used for anaesthesia.
- Oliver Wendell Holmes coined the term 'anaesthesia'.

Anesthetic agent	*Person associated with it*
1. Ether	Valeus Cordus
2. Chloroform	Simpson
3. Thiopentone (first intravenous anesthetic)	John Lundy
4. Cocaine (first local anesthetic)	Carl Koller

- First spinal anesthesia—given by August Beir.

  First epidural anesthesia—given by cathelin and Sicard.

  First endotracheal intubation—done by Ivan Magill.

  First clinical use of nitrous oxide—done by Humphry Davy.
- Colour code markings mentioned on vaporizers:

  Red – halothane
  Orange – enflurane
  Purple – isoflurane
  Yellow – sevoflurane

  Mnemonic: ROPY—**HE I**s Safe.
- **Methoxyflurane** is the only inhalational agent with boiling point more than water.

Anesthetic agent	*Boling point*	*Vapour pressure*
Ether	35°C	425 mm Hg
Halothane	50°C	243 mm Hg
Isoflurane	49°C	250 mm Hg
Nitrous oxide	-88°C	Gases
Methoxy flurane	105°C	23 mm Hg

- Methoxyflurane is the most potent inhalational agent and nitrous oxide is the least potent agent.

Anesthetic agent	*Minimun alveolar concentation (MAC)*
1. Methoxyflurane	0.16%
2. Halothane	0.74%
3. Isoflurane	1.15%
4. Sevoflurane	2.05%
5. Desflurane	6.0%
6. Nitrous oxide	104%

Anesthetic agent	*Blood gas partition coefficient*
1. Desflurane	0.42
2. Nitrous oxide	0.47
3. Sevoflurane	0.69
4. Isoflurane	1.38
5. Halothane	2.4
6. Methoxyflurane	15

- Induction is fastest with desflurane and slowest with methoxyflurane and so the recovery is fastest with desflurane.
- Fink effect (diffusion hypoxia) is seen towards the end of surgery, when nitrous oxide is closed the gradient reverses and the nitrous oxide from blood flow to alveoli replacing the oxygen causing hypoxia.
- Maximum depression of respiration—Enflurane. Maximum inhibition to ventilatory respouse—Halothane.

Maximum bronchodilatation in asthmatics—Halothane (Anaesthesia of choice).
Maximum bronchodilatation in non-asthmatics—Sevoflurane.
Maximum hypotension—Isoflurane (Agent of choice for controlled hypotension).

- Cardiovascular stability:
  Isoflurane > Desflurane >Sevoflurane > Halothane > Enflurane.
  So, isoflurane is the agent of choice for cardiac patients (except patients with myocardial ischemia) because of its minimum effect on baroreceptor reflex and maintenance of cardiac output.
- Heart is sensitized to adrenaline by:
  1. Halothane ***(AIPG '06)***
  2. Trielene.
  3. Cyclopropane.
  4. Chloroform.
  5. Enflurane.
- **Inhalational agents** are **fluorinated** to decrease their flammability.
- The nephrotoxicity produced by fluorinated agents is vasopressin resistant polyuric renal failure.
- Anesthetic agent with maximum analgesic properties is **trielene.**
- Metabolic Products of halothane are:
  1. Trifluoroacetic acid.
  2. Chloride.
  3. Bromide.
  4. Fluoride produced only under anaerobic conditions.
- Isoflurane—agent of choice for neurosurgery because rise in intracranial pressure is minimum and this rise

can be reversed with hyperventilation. It also decreases brain's oxygen consumption. It is also agent of choice for cardiac patients.

- Sevoflurane—agent of choice for induction in children because of its faster, pleasant and smooth induction with no significant systemic toxicity.
- Ether is the only agent (inhalational) which preserves ciliary activity.
- Cyclopropane—agent of choice of patients in shock.
- Propofol—agent of choice for total intravenous anesthesia and for induction in susceptible individuals for malignant hyperthermia.
- Dibucaine is the most potent, most toxic and longest acting local anesthesia.
- 2-chloroprocaine is the shortest acting local anesthetic agent.
- Procaine has the maximum vasodilating properties among other local anesthetic agents.
- Image magnification may be minimized by using a long cone.
- Foreshortening and elongation are produced by incorrect vertical angulation.
  1. When a patient is positioned for a panoramic exposure with the chin tilted too far upward, a reverse occlusal plane curve or a reverse smile line Mandibular structures look narrower and maxillary structures look wider (looks like a frown).
  2. Chin tilted too far downward:
     - An exaggerated smile line (big smile) i.e. occusal plane shows and excessive upward curve.
     - Sever interproximal overlapping, anterior teeth appear very distorted.

- Crescent-shaped radiolucent marks on dental radiograph is due to overbent films (cracked emulsion).
- The most common digital image receptor is charge-coupled device (CCD). It is a solid state receptor with a silicon chip embedded in it. It is the electronic circuit in the silicon chip that is sensitive to X-rays.
- Storage phosphor digital imaging system uses a reversible imaging plate instead of a sensor to record the image.
- Digital radiography requires less radiation because the sensor is more sensitive to X-rays than the film of traditional radiography. The sensor is used in place of film in digital radiography. Radiation exposure to the patient is reduced by 50-80% with digital radiography.
- The differentiating feature of bleeding in black eye and due to fracture of orbit is posterior limit of subconjunctival haemorrhage can be seen in black eye.
- Traumatic telecanthus is associated with naso-ethmoidal injury.
- There are chances of injuring facial artery and vein while doing circum-mandibular wiring.
- Epiphora results due to blockage of nasolacrimal duct.
- Entonox is a mixture of 50% N_2O and 50% O_2.
- **ECG changes** is first observed when level of lignocaine is more than 5-6 μg/ml.
- The vasoconstrictor of choice in patients suffering from hypertension is felypressin.
- Bulls eye appearance is seen in radiograph of lingually placed mandibular 3rd molar.

- Extraction of teeth is absolutely contraindicated in central hemangioma.
- Extraction of a tooth during acute infection helps drainage and relieves pain if proper antibiotic is given and its adequate blood level is reached. ***(BHU '06)***
- Local anesthesia with adrenaline is absolutely contraindicated in patients with untreated hyperthyroidism.
- The ideal treatment for fracture of the angle of mandible is plating to the convex surface of the mandible at its lower border.
- A patient with unfavourable fracture of the angle is best treated by open reduction with rigid bone fixation. ***(AIPG '94)***
- Dautery procedure is a treatment modality for repeated dislocation of the condyle.
- Nasal antrostomy is usually done through inferior meatus. ***(AIPG '98)***
- An empty cavity in the mandible with no lining is most likely to be idiopathic bone cavity. ***(AIIMS '99)***
- **Punch biopsy** is used in mass **screening** of **cancer patients**.
- Packing of wounds with iodoform gauze permits healing by secondary intention.
- Healing after flap surgery is by primary intention.
- Mepivacaine is the least vasodilating local anaesthesia.
- Waldron's method or Partsch II operation is marsupialization followed by enucleation of cysts.
- Temperature range of cryosurgery is –20°C to –180°C.

Liquid nitrogen, liquid carbon dioxide or nitrous oxide are used in cryosurgery.

- Normal value of hematocrit is 45 while for elective surgery, the minimal acceptable value is 30. *(AIIMS '93)*
- The best treatment for fractures of mandible with full complement of teeth is closed reduction with intermaxillary fixation.
- A patient with maxillofacial trauma requires **60 mmol** of potassium and **100 mmol** of sodium daily. *(AIIMS '04)*
- The area of the brain that is the 'last one' to be depressed by general anaesthesia agents is **medulla oblongata**. *(BHU '06)*
- Incisional biopsy of an ulcer is taken from the edge of the lesion along with normal tissues. *(BHU '06)*
- **Basal cell carcinoma** has no tendency for metastasis. *(BHU '06)*
- Most common route for metastasis of oral cancer is by **lymphatic spread.**
- The purpose of taping the eyes shut before surgery is to prevent corneal abrasion.
- Drug of choice in management of the acute allergic reaction involving bronchospasm and hypotension is adrenaline. *(BHU '06)*
- Keen's approach is an intraoral approach for reduction of zygomatic bone/arch fracture.
- **Sausage-string appearance** is seen in the sialogram of sialodochitis.

- Symptoms indicating the correct level of sedation after diazepam administration is 50% ptosis of eyelids, blurring of vision, slurring of speech (**Verill's sign**). *(AIIMS May '06)*
- N_2O–O_2 sedation is contraindicated in:
  1. Emphysema.
  2. Emotional instability.
  3. Upper respiratory obstruction.
- Line of withdrawal of a tooth is mainly determined by the root pattern of the tooth.
- Postage stamp method is a method of bone removal used in transalveolar extraction.
- Patients presently or having had a recent course of steroids for longer than 1 week should be given 200 mg hydrocortisone orally the day before surgery, 100 mg orally postoperatively, 100 mg orally the day after surgery, with return to a regular dose the second day postoperatively.
- Maximum dose of adrenaline in normal patients is **0.2 mg.**
- Maximum dose of adrenaline in cardiac patients is **0.04 mg.**
- A person with mucormycosis is generally treated with Amphotericin B.
- Radiation induced thyroid cancer is due to somatic radiation.
- Quality of the X-ray is governed by kilovoltage peak.
- Most sensitive phase in cell division to radiation is G_2 phase. *(AIPG '94)*
- Mirror image type of bone loss pattern is seen in localized juvenile periodontitis.

- Bitewing radiographs are taken first during full mouth survey of an adult.
- Herring bone pattern is produced when X-ray films are exposed in reversed direction.
- Fog on X-ray film is due to overdevelopment of film, improper safe lighting, deteriorated film, light leaks and use of contaminated fixing and developing solutions.
- Double exposure of X-ray film results in blurring.
- **Fingerprint contamination** of film leads to dark spots or lines.
- Film packet reversed in mouth results in light radiograph.
- Yellowish brown staining of 10PA X-ray film is due to insufficient washing. ***(AIIMS 2k)***
- The operator should stand at least 6 feet from the patient at an angle of 90 to 135 degrees to the central ray of the X-ray beam while taking X-ray.
- Hyperbaric oxygen uses 100% oxygen at 2 atmospheric pressure.
- The first step when initiating cardiopulmonary Resuscitation is establishment of unresponsiveness.
- **Thrombocytopenia** is the most common cause of hemorrhagic disorders.
- Alloplastic grafts are inert, man-made synthetic materials.
- Malocclusion is the most common pathognomonic sign of a mandibular fracture.
- The optimum site for IV sedation for an outpatient is the median cephalic vein.

- Class II lever is used during tooth extractions.
- Highest incidence of fractures occurs in young males between the ages of 15 and 24 years.
- Dead space in a wound is any area that remains devoid of tissue after closure of the wound. It usually fills in with blood which creates hematoma with a high potential for infection.
- Adrenal cortex secrete 20 mg of hydrocortisone daily.

CHAPTER TWO

Conservative Dentistry

- Prevention and control of dental carries is the foremost objective of restorative dentistry.
- The amount of translucency of enamel is related to variations in the degree of calcification and homogeneity.
- Enamel tufts are hypomineralized structures of enamel rods and inter-rod substance that project between adjacent groups of enamel rods from dentino enamel junction.
- The dentinoenamel junction is a hypermineralized zone. It is scalloped in outline with the crest of the waves penetrating toward the enamel.
- The course of the dentinal tubules is a slight s-curve in the tooth crown, but the tubules are straighter in the incisal ridges, cusps, and root areas.
- In dead tracts, the dentinal tubules are empty and thus appear black when ground sections of dentin are viewed microscopically with transmitted light. (Mnemonic: **D**ead **t**ract : **d**ark, **t**ransmitted light)
- Smear layer of dentin is composed of denatured collagen, hydroxyapatite, and other cutting debris.
- Embrasures are V-shaped spaces that originate at the proximal contact areas between adjacent teeth.

- Posselt's diagram record the mandible's motion.
- Root caries lesions tend to be U-shaped in cross-section.
- The primary goal of a caries prevention program is to reduce the number of cariogenic bacteria.
- Frequent ingestion of foods containing sucrose provides a stronger potential for colonization by streptococcus mutans, enhancing the caries potential of the plaque.
- Xylitol is a natural five-carbon sugar obtained from birch trees. It keeps the sucrose molecule from binding with streptococcus mutans. S. mutans cannot ferment xylitol. Thus, xylitol helps arrest dentinal caries.
- Metallic mercury vapour can be inhaled and absorbed through the alveoli in the lungs at 80% efficiency.

Absorption efficiency of mercury

	Skin	*Lungs*	*Gastrointestinal tract*
1. Organic	—	—	95-98% *(AIPG '06)*
2. Inorganic	—	80%	7%
3. Elemental	—	80%	0.01%

- Methyl mercury is an organic compound of mercury.
- Average half-life of mercury is **55 days** for transport through the body to the point of excretion. ***(AIIMS '06)***
- Threshold limit value for exposure to mercury vapour is 50 $\mu g/m^3$.
- The detection limit for mercury in water is approximately 0.02 µg/L.
- The principal feature of a sealant required for success is adequate retention.

- The ideal time to apply pit and fissure sealants is soon after occlusal surfaces erupt into the oral environment.
- Barium, zinc, boron, zirconium, yttrium have been used to produce radiopacity in the filler particles of composites.
- The most important clinical requirements of luting agents are flow, wetting, and film thickness. To produce a film thickness of less than 25 μm, cement particles of 5 μm or less is used.
- To treat dentin hypersensitivity, CO_2 laser irradiation, dentin adhesives, antibacterial agents, aldehydes, resin suspensions, fluoride rinses, fluoride varnishes, calcium phosphate, potassium nitrate, and oxalates are used.
- Gingival margin trimmer has four number code cutting instrument formula.
- Silicon carbide is the most commonly used abrasive for sandpapers.
- Aluminium oxide is used to manufacture sharpening stones.
- Spoon excavtors and discoids are the most difficult instruments to sharpen on a flat stone.
- Rotary speed ranges:

Slow or Low	→ < 12,000 rpm
Intermediate/Medium	→ 12,000-200,000 rpm
Ultrahigh/High	→ > 200,000 rpm

- The most important design characteristic of a bur blade is **the rake angle.**
- Cutting effectiveness is the rate of tooth structure removal (mm/min or mg/sec).

- Cutting efficiency is the percentage of energy actually producing cutting.
- S.C. Barnum introduced the rubber dam in 1864.
- Fletcher introduced silicate cement, the first translucent filling material.
- **Wilson** and **Kent** developed glass ionomers in 1972.
- The CEREC system was the first commercially available CAD/CAM system developed for the rapid chairside design and fabrication of ceramic restorations.
- Optical impression is the step in which a scanning device is used to collect information about the shape of the tooth preparation and its relationship with the surrounding structures.
- According to the formula of golden proportion, a smile, when viewed from the front, considered to be esthetically pleasing if each tooth in that smile starting from the midline is approximately **60%** of the size of the tooth immediately mesial to it. The exact proportion of the smaller tooth to the larger tooth is 0.618. ***(AIIMS '06)***
- The main deleterious side effect of non-vital bleaching technique (Thermocatalytic technique and walking bleach technique) is cervical resorption.
- 35% H_2O_2 is used in thermocatalytic technique of bleaching.
- 10% to 15% carbamide peroxide (degrades into 3% H_2O_2 and 7% urea) is used in nightguard vital bleaching.
- 35% H_2O_2 is used in power bleaching (in-office vital bleaching technique).

- A window preparation protect the veneers from significant occlusal stress by preserving the lingual and incisal surfaces of the maxillary anterior teeth.
- Porcelain veneers are etched with hydrofluoric acid.
- Dark discolorations of teeth are best treated with etched porcelain veneers.
- The universal matrix system was designed by **B.R.Tofflemire**. The thickness of matrix band available are 0.002 inch and 0.0015 inch.
- The primary function of the matrix is to restore anatomic contours and contact areas.
- In quadrant dentistry, when a quadrant of amalgam tooth preparation is planned, each rotary or hand instrument should be used on every tooth where it is needed before being exchanged.
- The most frequently used pin type is the small self threading pin.
- In 1966 Going described the pin-retained amalgam restoration using self-threading pin. The diameter of the prepared pinhole is 0.0015 to 0.004 inch smaller than the diameter of the pin.
- In1958 Markley described a technique for restoring teeth amalgam and cemented pins—using threaded stainless steel pins. Pinholes prepared are 0.001 to 0.002 inch larger than the diameter of the pin.
- 1966, Goldstein described friction locked pin. Pinhole prepared is 0.001 inch smaller than the diameter of the pin. The pins are tapped into place, retained by the resiliency of the dentin, and 2 to 3 times more retentive than cemented pin.

- **Self-threading** pin is the most retentive pin while **cemented pin** is the least retentive pin.
- As the number of pins increases, the strength of the amalgam restoration decreases.
- Retention is increased by placing pins in a non-parallel manner.
- As the diameter of the pin increases, the retention in dentin and amalgam increases.
- Pin extension into dentin and amalgam greater than 2 mm is contraindicated.
- One pin per missing axial line angle is used.
- The pinhole should be parallel to the adjacent external surface of the tooth.
- The pinhole should be positioned no closer than 0.5 to 1 mm to the dentinoenamel junction or no closer than 1 to 1.5 mm to the external surface of the tooth.
- Designs of Thread Made System are:

  Standard, self-shearing, two-in-one, link series, link plus.
- The gingival bevel of cast metal cavity should be 0.5 to 1 mm wide and should blend with the lingual secondary flare. The bevel results in 30-degree metal that is burnishable.
- Hand pressure is used for compaction of powdered gold while malleting is used for **compaction** of gold foil.
- If the nib diameter of the condenser is reduced by half, the compaction force in pounds per square inch is four times greater.

- Debridement is the last step of cavity preparation. *(BHU '06)*
- Rounding of axiopulpal line angle increases the fracture resistance of the restoration. ***(AIPG '06)***
- Primary teeth and fluoride treated teeth require longer time for acid etching due to the presence of less enamel prism.
- The main ingredient of dental ceramics is feldspar.
- **Refractive Index** of feldspathic porcelain is 1.504.
- For better bonding of ceramic restorations, etching is done with hydrofluoric acid or phosphoric acid.
- **Taggart** gave the lost wax technique of casting.
- **Sprue** former diameter is equal to the maximum thickness of the pattern. The main purpose of frozen slab technique of mixing zinc phosphate cement is to prolong the working time.
- Initiations and Achivators in composites:

Chemically activated composite		*UV light activated*	*Visible light cured composites*
Initiatiors :	Benzoyl Peroxide (diketone)	Benzoin methyl ether	Camphoroquinone (diketone)
Activators :	N.N. dimethyl toluidine (Tertiary amine)	UV light of wavelength 360 nm	Visible light of wave-length 460-480 nm

- BISGMA was developed by Bowen.
- The coupling agent used in composite resin is organosilane.
- Classification of composite resin according to filler particle size:

Type of composite resin	Filler particle size
1. Macrofilled	8-12 μm
2. Small particle	1-5 μm
3. Microfilled	0.04-0.4 μm
4. Hybrid	0.6-1 μm

- Types of curing lamps for light activated composites:
  1. Light Emitting Diodes (LED) lamps:
     It emits radiation only in the blue part of visible spectrum i.e. 440-480 nm.
  2. Quartz-Tungsten Halogen Lamps (QTH Lamps):
     It emits radiation of wavelength 400-500 nm.
  3. Plasma Arc Curing Lamps (PAC Lamps):
     It uses xenon gas to produce plasma. After filtration to remove heat wavelength of 400-500 nm is emitted.
  4. Argon Laser Lamps:
     It produce a wavelength of 490 nm.
     Quartz-Tungsten Halogen Lamps is the most widely used light source.
- Acid etching technique was first used by **Buonocore.**
- The most commonly used etchant is 37% phosphoric acid. Concentrations greater than 50% result in the formation of a monocalcium phosphate monohydrate that inhibits further dissolution while concentration below 30% results in dicalcium phosphate dihydrate that cannot be easily removed.
- Father of the dental amalgam is G.V. Black.
- The silver amalgam restoration lasts for about 15 years if manipulation is proper.
- Finishing of composite restoration is done 5 minutes after curing.

- Finishing of high copper single composition alloys is done 1 hour after restoration.
- For low copper alloys finishing is done 24 hours after restoration.
- Carving of amalgam restoration is usually done 15-20 minutes after restoration though it can be done immediately.
- Threshold level value for the amount of mercury vapours in blood and in urine are 3 mg/litre and < 7 mg/litre respectively.
- Death occurs if mercury content is ≥ 4 mg/kg weight of the person.
- Flouride containing $ZnPO_4$ cements are made by adding small percentage of stannous fluoride.
- Silicate cement is contraindicated in mouth breathers because the cement gets dried and becomes powdery and opaque.
- Eugenol in zinc oxide eugenol is a solvent for resins. Hence zinc oxide eugenol is contraindicated to use as a base for composite resins.
- Zinc polycarboxylate cement was introduced by Dr. Smith. It was the first dental cement which is adhesive to tooth structure.
- The compounds of fluoride used in glass ionomer cements are aluminium fluoride, calcium fluoride and sodium fluoride.
- Dr. McLean developed glass cermet cement in which silver particles are bonded to glass powder particles by fusion.

- **Dr. Siemens** developed miracle mix GIC in which spherical amalgam alloy powder is mixed with type II GIC powder.
- Setting expansion of zinc containing amalgam alloys occur after 3 to 5 days when there is moisture contamination. Hydrogen gas is produced by electrolytic action of zinc and water. This hydrogen collects within the restoration creating internal pressure and expansion of the restoration.

$$H_2O + Zn \rightarrow ZnO + H_2 \text{ (gas)}$$

- The reduction of cusp tends to decrease **retention form.**
- Cutting instrument formula:
  It can be a three or four numbers code.

  First number indicates the width of the blade in tenths of a millimeter.

  Second number of four number code indicates the cutting edge angle measured from a line parallel to the long axis of the instrument in clockwise centigrades. The angle is expressed as a percent of 360°. This number should always **exceed 50**. If the edge is perpendicular to the blade, this number is omitted.

  Third number indicates the blade length in millimeters.

  Fourth number indicates the blade angle, relative to the long axis of the handle in clockwise centigrade. This number should be **50 or less.**
- Angle former and gingival margin trimmer have four number code instrument formula.

Cutting instruments	Use
1. Ordinary hatchet excavators	Preparation of retentive areas and sharpening internal line angles particularly for direct gold restorations
2. Hoe excavator	Planing tooth preparation walls and forming line angles
3. Angle former	Sharpening line angles creation of retentive features in direction for gold restorations

- Gingival margin trimmer is used to produce bevel on gingival enamel margins of proximoocclusal prepartions.

  If second number is 90 to 100 = used on distal gingival margin

  If second number is 85 to 75 = used on mesial gingival margin

  100 and 75 pairs – for inlay and onlay to make steep gingival bevels

  90 and 85 pairs – for amalgam preparations to make bevels that decline slightly.

- Steps of tooth (cavity) preparation:
  1. Outline form and initial depth.
  2. Primary resistance form.
  3. Primary retention form.
  4. Convenience form.
  5. Removal of infected dentin or old restorative material if indicated.
  6. Pulp protection if indicated.
  7. Secondary resistance and retention forms.
  8. Finishing of external walls.
  9. **Cleaning, inspecting and sealing.** ***(BHU '06)***

- Internal and external angles within the tooth preparation are slightly rounded or coved to prevent stress concentration from masticatory forces at these line angles.
- Rounding of external angles (eg. axiopulpal line angle) increases resistance to fracture of amalgam and porcelain by reducing stress concentration. ***(AIPG '06)***
- Retention in Class I and Class II amalgam restoration is provided by converging external tooth walls.
- Retention in Class III and Class V (conventional) is provided by retention coves or grooves in the dentinal wall since the external walls diverge outwardly to provide strong enamel margins.
- The cavosurface bevel of tooth preparation for gold alloy castings should be 30 to 40 degree.
- Gingival bevel of a casting should be 30 degree to provide a sliding, lap fit that improves adaptation of a metal to tooth.
- **Bowen** introduced **composites**.
- **The configuration factor (c-factor)** is the ratio of bonded surfaces to the unbonded, free surfaces in a tooth preparation. It affects the polymerization shrinkage of composite materials. The higher the C-factor, the greater is the potential for bond disruption from polymerization effects.
- Internal stresses due to high disruptive contraction forces in composite restorations can be reduced by:
  1. Slow on soft start polymerization instead of high intensity light curing.
  2. Incremental additions to reduce the effects of polymerization shrinkage.

3. Use of stress-breaking liner, such as filled dental adhesive or resin modified glass ionomer.

- Direction of polymerization shrinkage for self cured composite material is towards the center of the mass. It helps to maintain marginal adaptation to prevent microleakage.
- A V-shaped gap (contraction gap) is formed between the root and the composite when the tooth preparation is extended onto the root surface with composite restorations. This gap occurs due to greater force of polymerization shrinkage of the composite than the initial bond strength of the composite to the dentin of the root (no marginal enamel).
- In tooth preparation of a proximal surface of an anterior tooth (i.e. Class III or Class IV) for composite restoration, the entry into the tooth is generally done from lingual side. Advantages for lingual approach are:
  1. The facial enamel is conserved for enhanced esthetics.
  2. Some unsupported, but not friable, enamel may be left on the facial wall of a Class III or Class IV preparation.
  3. Discoloration or deterioration of the restoration is less visible.
- The axial wall of Class III composite tooth preparation is convex outwardly both incisogingivally and faciolingually.
- The outline form of Class IV composite restoration is prepared by making the walls as much as possible perpendicular or parallel to the long axis of the tooth. This provides greater resistance to biting forces.

- The primary retention form of Class IV composite restoration is provided by the micromechanical bonding of the composite to the enamel and dentin.
- Gingival retention groove in Class IV tooth preparation extends the length of the gingival floor and slightly up the facioaxial and linguoaxial line angles.
- The outline form of Class V tooth preparation is dictated by the extent of caries defect, or old restorative material indicated for replacement.
- The axial wall of Class V composite tooth preparation is convex outward mesiodistally and sometimes occlusogingivally.
- **Dicor restorations** are made using a lost-wax method and **centrifugal** casting process.
- The most likely cause for not fitting of inlay or onlay restoration into the tooth preparation is **overcontoured proximal surface.**
- Chairside etching of ceramic inlays and onlays is done with a 2 minute application of 10% hydrofluoric acid on the internal surfaces of the inlay/onlay.
- Cusp reduction decreases retention form because of decreasing the height of the vertical walls.
- Excavators have four subdivisions:
  1. Ordinary hatchet.
  2. Hoes.
  3. Angle formers.
  4. Spoon excavators.

Chisels are used for cutting enamel. It may be:

1. Bin-angle —Planing of cavity wall
2. Wedelstaedt —Planing of cavity wall
3. Enamel hatchet —Cutting of enamel
4. Gingival margin trimmer —beveling of gingival margin

- The **Class III tooth preparation** for gold restoration was first described by **Ferrier**.
- The Class V tooth preparation for direct gold restoration is trapezoidal. This outline form satisfy both esthetic needs and requirements for retention and convenience forms in the treatment of lesions in the gingival third.
- The axial wall of Class III tooth preparation for gold restoration is flat faciolingually and incisogingivally.
- Lingual 'slot' type of preparation with rounded internal line angles is made when powdered gold pellets is used for lingual approach Class III restorations.
- 'Shoe' refers to the minimal or partial coverage of the cusp by means of a finishing bevel on the crest of the cusp.
- **Amalgam adhesives** seal the dentin with an acid-resistant layer of resin-reinforced dentin called the hybrid layer. This is a multistepped procedure that involves applying an etchant, primer, and adhesive to the prepared tooth surface. Adhesives used with amalgam is self-curing.
- The matrix for the **occluso-lingual amalgam** restoration is referred to as the **Barton matrix**.

Rubber dam

1. S.C. Barnum introduced the rubber dam.
2. The bow of the retainer (except the No. 212, which is applied after the rubber dam is in place) is tied with dental floss to allow retrieval of the retainer or its broken parts if they are accidentally swallowed or aspirated. ***(AIPG '94)***
3. Retainer is usually not required for anterior tooth, except for the cervical retainer for Class V restorations.

Contd.

Contd.

4. Rubber dam is available in the following thickness:

Thin	–	0.006 inch (0.15 mm)
Medium	–	0.008 inch (0.2 mm)
Heavy	–	0.010 inch (0.25 mm)
Extra heavy	–	0.012 inch (0.30 mm)
Special heavy	–	0.014 inch (0.35 mm)

5.

Region or tooth of operation	**Region of isolation**
1. Incisors and mesial surfaces of canines	First premolar to first premolar
2. Canine other than mesial surfaces	First molar to the opposite lateral incisor
3. Premolars	Two teeth distally and anteriorly the opposite lateral incisor
4. Molars	As far distally as possible and anteriorly the opposite lateral incisor

- For **endodontic** therapy only the tooth to be treated is isolated. *(AIPG '06)*
- Minimum of three teeth is recommended for isolation.
- The distance between holes is equal to the distance from the center of one tooth to the center of the adjacent tooth, measured at the level of the gingival tissue. It is approximately ¼ inch (6.3 mm). *(AIPG '06)*
- The first holes punched (after the identification hole) when the rubber dam is applied to the maxillary teeth are for the central incisors.
- The first hole punched (after the identification hole) when the rubber dam is applied to the maxillary teeth are for **the central incisors.**

- The first hole punched (after the identification hole) when the rubber dam is applied to the mandibular teeth is for the posterior anchor tooth that is to receive the retainer.
- The first step of placement of rubber dam is testing and lubricating the proximal contacts.
- The first step in removal of rubber dam is cutting the septal rubber.
- The jaws of the retainers used on primary and young permanent teeth is directed more gingivally because the anchor tooth's height of contour is below the crest of the gingival tissue or because of short clinical crowns.
- The S.S. white No. 27 retainer is recommended for primary teeth while the Ivory No. W14 retainer is recommended for young permanent teeth.

ADDITIONAL HIGH YIELD FACTS

- Mesial and distal wall of class V cavity depends on direction of enamel rods while the outline form depends on extension of the caries. ***(AIPG '02)***
- Gingival extension for a restoration is at least 3 mm above the alveolar crest. ***(AIPG '02)***
- Eugenol can be replaced in the zinc oxide euginol cement by ortho-ethoxy acid. ***(AIIMS '99)***
- Resin modified glass ionomer is designed to provide rapid setting to minimize cement acidity allowing early finishing.
- The property of amalgam that makes it undesirable to bevel occlural margins of an amalgam cavity preparation is its brittleness. ***(AIIMS 2K)***

- The discoloured corroded superficial layer frequently seen to the surface of amalgam restoration is most likely a sulfide. *(AIPG '91)*
- **Colour dye detector** is used for differentiating between affected and effected dentin.
- The most important cause for marginal failure of amalgam restoration is increased creep. *(AIPG '91)*
- Polishing agent for amalgam is tin oxide/zinc oxide.
- The occlusal clearance of an onlay is best detected by wax chew in. *(AIPG 2K)*
- Cast gold alloy is polished by rouge.
- Reverse bevel or counter bevel are given to counteract oblique forces. *(AIPG '94)*
- Pain and sensitivity in a tooth with onlay after 4 months is due to supra occlusion. *(AIIMS '97)*
- Crucible indicated for casting base metal alloys is quartz crucible while for casting gold alloys is carbon crucible. *(AIPG '04)*
- Titanium casting is done by using copy Milling system.
- Beilby layer is a molecular disorganized structure surface on a highly polished metal surface.
- Porosity in porcelain at condensation stage depends on shape and size of particle. *(AIPG 2K)*
- Instrument used to plane buccoproximal and linguoproximal walls in class II cavity is enamel hatchet. *(AIPG '96)*
- A proximal carious lesion in a radiograph is smaller than clinically. *(BHU '06)*
- The thickness of the band material used for class II restoration is 0.002 inch. *(AIPG '96)*

- Lethal form of mercury is organic form (i.e. ethyl or methyl mercury).
- Spheroiding is the tendency of amalgam to become rounded in plastic stage.
- The property of gold that is not affected by cold working is modulus of elasticity.
- Composite resin is best polished by aluminium oxide.
- **Sprue l**ength and **l**ocalized shrinkage porosity have direct relationship.
- **Sprue** diameter and subsurface porosity have direct relationship.
- The boiling point of mercury is—**356.90°C.**
  Freezing point of mercury is **–38.87°C.**
- Creep values:

Low-Copper Amalgam	–	0.8 to 8.0 %
High-Copper Amalgam	–	0.4 to 0.1%

- Bond strength to etched enamel range from 16 Mpa to 22 Mpa.

CHAPTER THREE

Endodontics

CLINICAL DIAGNOSTIC METHODS

1. The submandibular lymph nodes are involved when the posterior teeth are infected. Infection of the lower anterior teeth cause swelling of the submental lymph nodes.
2. Loss of cancellous bone is detectable by radiograph when 6.6% of the mineral content of the cortical bone is lost.
3. The objective of electric pulp testing is to stimulate a pulpal response by subjecting the tooth to an increasing degree of electric current.
4. Application of CO_2 snow (–78°C) or Frigident spray (–50°C) is the test of choice for pulp vitality on teeth with full coverage restorations.
5. Ethyl chloride is used in cold testing.
6. A positive tooth vitality response of 98.7% is produced with dichloro-difluoro methane (DDM).
7. Excitation of the "A delta" nerve fibres in the pulp causes sharp, piercing and lancinating type of pulpal pain.
8. Excitation of the "C" nerve fibres causes dull, boring, gnawing, and excruciating type of pulpal pain.

9. Percussion, palpation, mobility, and depressibility are tests of the periodontium.
10. Periapical osteofibrosis (ossifying periapical fibroma, periapical rarefying osteitis, ossifying fibroma, cementoma, cementoblastoma, osseous dysplasia) appear radiolucent on the radiograph. It is often delineated at the periphery by sclerotic bone.

Sterilisation of instruments

Instrument	*Sterilising method*
1. Burs	Autoclave, dry heat
2. Broaches, files, reamers	Hot salt sterilizes or glass bead sterilizer for 5 sec.
3. Absorbent points, cotton pellets	Hot salt or glass-bead sterilizer for 10 sec.
4. Dapper dishes	Tincture of thimerosal (merthiolate) followed by alcohol
5. Cement spatula	Heat flame
6. Blades of scissors	Alcohol and flaming
7. Glass slab	Tincture of thimerosal followed swabbing with alcohol
8. Gutta percha cones	5.2% sodium hypochlorite, H_2O_2
9. Silver cones	Bunsen flame, hot salt sterilizer for 5 sec.

- The temperature of glass bead in glass bead sterilizer is between 218°C (425°F) and 246°C (475°F).
- The hottest part of the salt bath or glass bead bath is along its outer rim.
- The size of glass bead is less than 1 mm in diameter.
- Trephination is the creation of surgical passage in the region of the root apex to provide a channel for the escape of pus and blood, to relieve the pressure of accumulated fluid or gas in the jaw bone.

- The gram-positive organisms found in root canals are streptococci, staphylococci, corynebacteria, yeasts.
- The gram-negative bacteria found in root canal are spirochetes neisseria, bacteroides, fusobacterium, pseudomonas, coliform bacteria.
- Bacteria enter the pulp through the crown or root following traumatic exposure of the pulp, from the periodontal tissue through exposed dentinal tubules, lateral and accessory canals, or apical and lateral foramina and by the lymphatic or hematogenous route.
- Anachoresis is defined as the localization of transient bacterial in the blood into an inflamed area, such as a traumatized or inflamed pulp.

ORAL EMBRYOLOGY

- The dental pulp developed at about **6th week of uterine life.**
- Hertwig's epithelial root sheath determines the size and shape of the root of the tooth.
- In multirooted teeth, the epithelial diaphragm guides the formation of the furca, roots, root canals, and apical foramina.
- A defect in the epithelial root sheath, a failure in the induction of dentinogenesis, or the presence of a small blood vessel produces a gap that results in the formation of an accessory canal.
- Cementocytes receive their nutrients from the periodontal ligament.
- Cementum is deposited in a thin layer at the cemento-enamel junction to form a butt joint (30%), an overlap joint (60%) or a gap between cementum and enamel

(10%). This gap may produce cervical sensitivity, or it may predispose the tooth to cervical caries.

- Continued incremental deposition of cementum in the apical third maintains the length of the tooth, constricts the apical foramen, and deviates the apical foramen from the center of the apex.
- The plexus of Raschkow is located in the subodontoblastic zone of the coronal pulp. These sensory nerve fibres are myelinated.
- The **sympathetic** nerve fibres entering the dental pulp are unmyelinated.
- The completion of the apical foramen marks the end of pulp development and the beginning of secondary dentin formation by the pulp.
- The average volume of pulp space is 0.024 ml in permanent adult human teeth.
- In the coronal pulp, the odontoblasts are tall, columnar cells with a nucleus polarized toward the center of the pulp.
- The primary function of the odontoblasts is the production and deposition of dentin.
- The configuration of the dentinal tubules is 'S' shaped in the pulpal side due to crowding of odontoblasts producing more dentinal tubules.
- The dentinal tubules are conical in shape, with a 2.5 μm mean diameter in the pulpal wall and a 0.9 μm mean diameter in the dentinoenamel or dentinocemental junction, because of the deposition of the peritubular dentin.
- Secondary dentin can be differentiated from primary dentin by the sharp bending of the tubules producing a line demarcation.

- Reparative dentin is formed due to noxious stimuli such as caries, operative procedures, abrasion, erosion, or trauma.
- The **demarcation zone** between secondary and reparative dentin is called the **calciotraumatic line**.
- The cell-free zone, or zone of Weil is located centrally to the odontoblast zone. The zone of Weil is more prominent in the coronal pulp.
- The main constituent of the pulp is ground substance which is composed of proteoglycans or mucopoly-saccharides like hyaluronic acid, chondroitin sulfate, dermatan sulfate, and heparin sulfate; glycoproteins and water.
- The function of fibroblasts is production of ground substance and collagen fibres.
- An average intrapulpal pressure of approximately 10 mm Hg is produced by the presence of interstitial fluid in the pulpal cavity.
- An increase in intrapulpal pressure to 13 mm Hg during inflammatory changes causes reversible changes in the pulp, but increase to 35 mm Hg produce irreversible changes.
- 80% of the nerves of the pulp are C-type fibres and 20% are A delta fibres. The C fibres are unmyelinated and have diameter of 0.3 to 1.2 μm and conduction velocity of 0.4 to 2 m/sec. The A delta fibres are myelinated and have diameter of 2 to 5 μm and conduction velocity of 6 to 30 m/sec.
- **Dentin sensitivity** is caused by the excitation of **A-delta fibres**.
- With advancing age, the fibroblasts are reduced in size and numbers, but the collagen fibres are increased in

number and in size probably because of the decrease in the collagen solubility and turnover.

- Acellular cementum is deposited first against the dentin and it covers the cervical and middle thirds of the roof.
- Cementum is more resistant to bone because of its avascularity.
- The periodontal ligament is thinner at the rotational.
- Symphathetic nerves accompany the arterial blood vessels in the periodontal ligament.
- With advancing age, the width of the periodontal ligament is reduced.

DISEASES OF THE DENTAL PULP AND PERIRADICULAR TISSUES

- **Cracked tooth syndrome** can be visualized by **fibreoptic transillumination.**
- Barodontalgia or aerodontalgia is observed in altitudes of 5,000 feet to 10,000 feet or above.
- W.D. Miller suggested that bacteria is the cause of inflammation in the pulp.
- Internal resorption is called pink spot and it represents the granulation tissue showing through the resorbed area of the crown.
- Phoenix abscess is an acute exacerbation of a chronic lesion.
- Tooth is vital in cementoma.
- About 75% of all periradicular cysts occur in maxilla and about 25% occur in the mandible.

- The distribution of cysts in the maxilla is:

Incisors	–	62%
Canine	–	7%
Premolars	–	20%
Molars	–	11%

- The distribution of periradicularcysts in the mandible is:

Incisors	–	16%
Canine	–	2%
Premolars	–	34%
Molars	–	48%

- Condensing osteitis is a mild irritation from pulpal disease that stimulates osteoblastic activity in the alveolar bone. It appears as radiopaque in the radiograph.

PREPARATION, DISINFECTION AND OBTURATION OF THE ROOT CANAL

- The fourth canal in the maxillary first molar is located palatal to the mesiobuccal orifice.
- Barbed broaches are available in a variety of sizes, from triple extra fine (XXXF) to extra coarse (XC).
- A 50% dilution of 5.2% solutions of sodium hypochlorite (Clonox or Purex) with distilled water gives a solution of 2.6% sodium hypochlorite. Sodium hypochlorite contains about 5% of available chlorine.
- Alternating solutions of 3% H_2O_2 and 5.2% sodium hypochlorite (NaOCl) produce effervescent reaction.
- Compressed air is not used for drying the root canal because tissue emphysema may result if an air bubble penetrates the periapical tissues.

- When 2 root canals are present in a single root, two length determination radiographs are taken, one at the normal angulation, the other at a 20° mesial or distal horizontal angulation.
- **Step-back method** is also known as **telescopic preparation of the root canal.**
- Engine driven instruments:
  1. The giromatic handpiece activates a stainless steel barbed broach or reamer in the root canal through a 90° reciprocating arc at a speed up to 1000 cycles/min.
  2. The Racer contra-angle handpiece uses a standard file and oscillates the file in the root canal.
- Power driven instruments:
  1. Gates Glidden drills has a long, thin shaft ending in a flame-shaped head, with a safe tip to guard against perforations. It is used in step-back preparation.
  2. The Peeso reamer has long, sharp flutes connected to a thick shaft.
- Ultrasonic instruments consist of a piezoelectric ceramic unit that generates ultrasonic waves, which activate a magnetostrictive stack handpiece. The handpiece holds a K-file on activation produces movements of the shaft of the file between 0.001 and 0.004 inch at a frequency of 20,000 to 25,000/sec.
- Ethylene diaminotetra-acetic acid was introduced by Nygoard-Ostby. It functions by forming a calcium-chelate solution with the calcium ion of dentin. The dentin becomes more friable.
- EDTAC is 15% solution of EDTA with 0.84 g of bactericide cetavlon added to it. It has pH of about 7.3.

- EDTA demineralizes dentin to a depth of 20 to 30 μ in 5 min.
- Stewart developed R-C prep which is a combination of EDTA and urea peroxide.
- K-file is first inserted into the root canal through the access cavity with a slight wiggling motion.
- The tip angle of an endodontic instrument is 75±15°.

Endodontic instruments	*Blanks from which they are made up of*
1. K-reamer	– Triangular blank
2. K-file	– Square blank
3. K-flex file	– Diamond shaped blank
4. Hedstroem file	– Round blank (spiral flutes)
5. Unifile	– Round blank (double helix)

- Aqueous solution of para-chlorophenol penetrates deeper into the dentinal tubules than camphorated chlorophenol.
- N2 contains para formaldehyde as its main ingredient is both an intracanal medicament and a sealer. Its actions dissipate in about a week to 10 days.
- The disinfected action of the halogens is inversely proportional to their atomic weights.
- Quaternary ammonium compounds cling to the microorganism because the former is positively charged while the latter is negatively charged.
- Cutting efficiency of the endodontic instruments follow in the order: Hedstroem file > K-flex file.
- Triangular-blanked instruments cut 2.5 times more efficiently than square blank instruments.
- Culture media for micro-organisms present in root canals are:

1. Infusion broth with 0.1% agar.
2. Trypticase soy broth with 0.1% agar.
3. Thioglycollate.
4. Glucose ascites broth.

- More than 48 hours or preferable 96 or more hours should be allowed between taking the culture and filling the root canal.
- The function of a root canal filling is to obturate the canal and eliminate all portals of entry between the periodontium and the root canal.
- A root canal is obturated when:
  1. Tooth is asymptomatic.
  2. Root canal is reasonably dry.
  3. After obtaining a negative culture.
  4. After closure of an existing sinus tract.
- Bowman introduced gutta-percha cones.
- Compositon of gutta perca cones:

Gutta-percha (matrix)	–	20%
Zinc oxide (filler)	–	66%
Heavy metal sulfates (radiopacifier)	–	11%
Waxes or resins (plasticizer)	–	3%

- The aged brittle gutta percha cone can be rejuvenated by momentary immersion in hot tap water (55°C) followed by instant cooling in cold tap water.
- Sorin and Oliet gave idea of rejuvenation of aged gutta-percha cone.
- Obturation technique indicated in post core crown is sectional method.
- Vertical-Condensation Method (Warm Gutta Percha) was introduced by Schilder.
- Compaction method was introduced by McSpadden.

- Chemically Plasticized Gutta Percha technique, Metal-core obturation method like silver-cone method, stainless steel file method are indicated in filling fine, tortuous canals.
- Stainless steel file method was introduced by Sampeck.
- Injection Technique of Obturating canals:
  1. Hydron—It is a polymer of hydroxy-ethyl-methacrylate and sets in 10 min.
  2. Thermoplasticized Gutt-Percha Method.
     Gutta percha is heated from 70° to 160°C depending on the method or material used.
- Composition of Grossman Cement:

Powder		*Parts*
1. **Z**inc oxide, reagent	–	42
2. **Stay**belite resin	–	27
3. **Bis**muth subcarbonate	–	15
4. **Bar**ium sulfate	–	15
5. **S**odium borate, anhydrous	–	1
Liquid		
1. Eugenol or oil of pimenta leaf (Mnemonic: **Z**.**Stay**Bis **B**afrS)		

- AH26 is an epoxy resin containing radiopaque bismuth oxide.
- Diaket is a polyvinyl resin (polyketone).
- AH26 and Diaket are root canal cements introduced by Schroeder and Scheufele respectively.

ADDITIONAL HIGH YIELD FACTS

- Tooth discolouration in systemic diseases and their colour of tooth.

1. Congenital porphyria	-	Red or purple
2. Hereditary opalescent dentin	-	Violaceous
3. Endemic fluorosis	-	Mottled brown
4. Erythroblastosis fetalis	-	Grayish brown
5. Jaundice	-	Brown

- **Green discoloration of teeth** associated with the Nasmyth's membrane occurs in children.
- Root fracture in the middle or coronal third of the root has poor prognosis because of the difficulty of immobilizing the tooth.
- Tests for pulp vitality is contraindicated for 6 to 8 weeks after the injury of a tooth.
- Avulsed tooth may be stored in milk for 6 hours; only 2 hours in saliva. Milk has no restorative effect when the periodontal ligament has already become dehydrated. ***(AIPG '06)***
- Intentional replantation means the removal of a tooth for the purpose of extra-oral endodontic treatment and the replacement of that tooth in its socket almost immediately. It is usually performed within 15 minute.
- Fauchard introduced intentional replantation.
- **The Achilles heel** of the endodontic implant is its apical seal.
- Orlay and Frank popularized the endodontic implants.
- Apexification is usually completed in 6 months to 2 years.
- Thermoplasticized gutta-percha technique is method of choice for obturation after apexification.
- The prognosis of apexification is guarded.
- The pulp chambers of the maxillary canine are the largest of any single-rooted teeth.

- The pulp chamber of the maxillary first molar is the **largest** in the dental arch.
- The mandibular central incisor is the smallest tooth in the arch.
- The mandibular first premolar is the transitional tooth between anterior and posterior teeth, and in anatomic structure it resembles both types of teeth.
- The prominent buccal cusp and the smaller lingual cusp give the crown of the mandibular first premolar about a 30° lingual tilt.
- Large pulp chamber is a characteristic of Neanderthal man.
- Taurodontism is due to lack of invagination of the epithelial root sheath during development. It occurs mainly in Eskimos.
- The addition of 0.5 to 1.0% zinc acetate accelerates the setting time of zinc-oxide eugenol and prevents its deformation.
- Specification of files and reamers:

Color code	*Number (size)*
Pink	6
Grey	8
Purple	10
White	15
Yellow	20
Red	25
Blue	30 ***(PGI '06)***
Green	35
Black	40

- Corticosteroid antibiotic paste is recommended in tooth in which over instrumentation has been done.

- Most important aspect of irrigation of canal is the volume of solution used.
- The length of the dowel should be 2/3rd the length of the root.
- Replacement resorption results in ankylosis.
- Palatal root of maxillary first molar is curved buccally. *(AIIMS '93)*
- Following endodontic treatment, repair of the previously damaged periapical tissue occurs in 6-12 months.
- The main objective of access cavity preparation is to obtain straight line access for proper instrumentation into the root canal. *(AIPG '06)*
- The most effective means of reducing microbes in root canal is complete debrediment through instrumentation.
- **Formocresol** produces tissue fixation and **coagulative necrosis.**
- For doing endodontic implants, the root canal is enlarged at least the size of a No. 60 instrument.
- Pain of dental origin is ipsilateral and never crosses midline i.e. on the opposite side.
- 40 mm long reamer is generally used for root canal preparation for doing endodontic implants.
- Accessory canals are most frequently found in the apical one third of the root. *(AIPG '96)*
- Two canals are most often seen in the root of mandibular first premolar.
- Internal resorption is due to chronic inflammation of pulp. *(AIPG '97)*

- The safest instrument for removing the pulp from the very fine canal is small K type file. *(AIPG '90)*
- For canal preparation of double-curved and dilacerated root canals a small Hedstroem file is used.
- K-file is the first instrument inserted into the root canal through the access cavity.
- Apicoectomy is contraindicated in extensive bone loss.
- Most of the failures of replanted tooth are due to external resorption. *(AIPG '03)*
- Exarticulation of teeth means avulsion. *(PGI '02)*
- **Pulse oximetry** is used in the determination of oxygen saturation. *(AIIMS May '06)*
- Laser Doppler flowmetry is a non-invasive method to measure the blood flow. *(AIIMS May '06)*
- In LASER root canal preparation, transformation of dentin into an ionized gas occurs. This is known as **plasma effect**.

Site of pain referral	*Tooth pulp causing pain*
1. Forehead region	Maxillary incisors
2. Nasolabial area	Maxillary canines, premolars
3. Temporal region	Maxillary second premolars
4. Ear	Mandibular molars
5. Mental region of mandible	Mandibular incisors, canines and premolars

- Reaming action produces a canal that is round in shape while a filing action produces a canal that is irregular in shape.

CHAPTER FOUR

Orthodontics

INTRODUCTION

- Le Foulon coined the term 'Orthodontia'.
- Edward H. Angle is considered the "Father of Modern Orthodontics". He developed the 'E' arch, the pin and the tube appliance, the ribbon arch appliance and the edgewise appliance.
- Pierre Fauchard, often called the "Father of Modern Dentistry" developed Bandelette now called the expansion arch. Bandelette is often considered the **first Orthodontic Appliance.**
- Dr. Norman W. Kingsley is considered as the pioneer in cleft palate treatment.
- Holly Broadbent and Hofrath independently developed cephalometric radiography.

GROWTH AND DEVELOPMENT

- Todd defined "Growth is an increase in size; development is progress towards maturity.
- Two important aspects of growth: Scammon's curve of growth and Cephalo—caudal gradient of growth.
- Points on Scammon' curve of growth:
  1. Lymphoid tissue proliferates rapidly and reaches almost 200% of adult size in late childhood.

2. Neural tissue reaches adult size by 6-7 years of age.
3. General tissue exhibit and "S" shaped curve.
4. After 10 years, 90% of maxillary growth is reached.

- Points on Cephalo-caudal gradient of growth:
  1. The head takes up about 50% of the total body length at about the third month of intrauterine development.
  2. At birth, the head is about 30% of body length.
  3. At birth the legs represent about one third of body length.
  4. Mandible tends to grow more and later than the maxilla.
- Dyes used for vital staining: Alizarin, Tetracycline, Lead acetate. Alizarin reacts strongly with calcium at sites where bone growth.
- John Hunter, English anatomist discovered alizarin.
- The fontanelles (loose connective tissues) allow a considerable amount of deformation of the skull at birth and this allow the relatively large head to pass through the birth canal.

THEORIES OF GROWTH

1. Genetic theory.
2. Sutural theory by Sicher.
3. Cartilaginous theory by James Scott.
4. Functional matrix theory by Melvin and Moss.
5. Multi-factorial theory by Van Limborgh.
6. Expanding 'V' principle by Enlow.
7. Counterpart principle by Enlow.

- Both intramembranous and endochondral bone formation takes place in **O**ccipital Bone, **M**andible, **T**emporal Bone, **S**phenoid Bone (Mnemonic: MOST).

- *Endochondral ossification:* Ethmoid bone, bones of cranial base.
- *Intramembranous ossification:* Maxilla, bones of cranial vault.

Bone	*No. of ossification center*
Occipital bone	7
Sphenoid bone	15
Temporal bone	11
Ethmoid bone	3

- Earliest evidence of formation of cranial base is seen in 4th-8th week of intra uterine development.
- The mid-palatal suture ossifies by 12-14 years.
- The Meckel's cartilage is derived from the first Branchial arch around 6th week of Intra uterine life.
- Classical conditioning of learning and development of behaviour is given by Ivan Pavlov.
- Operant Conditioning by **B.F. Skinner**.
- In Cognitive Development Theory, life is divided into:

1st stage:	Sensorimotor period	- birth to 2 years
2nd stage:	Preoperational period	- 2 to 7 years
3rd stage:	Concrete operational period	- 7 to puberty
4th stage:	Formal operations	- adolescence to adulthood

- Clefting of the lip occurs because of a failure of fusion between the median and lateral nasal processes and the maxillary prominence, which normally occurs in human during the sixth week of development.
- About 60% of individual with a cleft lip also have a cleft palate.

- Calcification of maxillary and mandibular central incisors begin at 14 week in utero.
- Calcification of maxillary and mandibular 1st molar begin at 15 week in utero.
- The suckling reflex and the infantile swallow normally disappear during the first year of life.
- **The total eruption path** of a first permanent molar is about **2.5 cm**.
- Dental age is determined by three characteristics:
  - Which teeth have erupted.
  - The amount of resorption of the roots of primary teeth.
  - The amount of development of the permanent teeth.
- Teeth usually emerge when three fourths of their roots are completed.
- The correlation coefficient between developmental status and chronologic age is about 0.8. The ability to predict one characteristic from another is equal to square of the correlation coefficient. So the probability that one could predict the developmental stage from knowing the chronologic age or vice-versa is $(0.8)^2 = 0.64$.
- Growth in width is completed first, then growth in length, and finally growth in height.
- The arch space for eruption of permanent mandibular 2nd and 3rd molars is gained by resorption of anterior border of ramus and apposition of posterior border of ramus of mandible. ***(AIIMS '06)***
- About one third of the Pierre Robin Syndrome patients have a defect in cartilage formation and is said to have stickler syndrome.

- **Acromegaly** patients have skeletal class III malocclusion.
- In **ectodermal dysplasia**, there is lack of development of the alveolar processes.
- The most common supernumerary tooth is mesiodens.
- Multiple supernumerary teeth are most often seen in cleidocranial dysplasia, which is characterized by missing clavicles, many supernumerary and unerupted teeth and failure of the succedaneous teeth to erupt.
- Ectopic eruption is most likely to occur in the eruption of maxillary first molars.
- The major reason for mesial movement of permanent teeth when a space opens up is due to mesial inclination, so that they erupt mesially as well as occlusally.
- When a primary first molar or canine is lost prematurely, there is distal drift of incisors to close the space and not by mesial drift of posterior teeth. This is due to: force from active contraction of **transseptal** fibres in the gingival, and pressures from the lips and checks.
- If a primary canine or first molar is lost prematurely on only one side, the permanent teeth drift distally only on that side, leading to asymmetry in the occlusion as well as tendency toward crowding.
- If thumbsucking created pressure against the teeth for 6 hours or more per day, it certainly could move teeth.
- Enlargement of the mandibular gonial angles takes place with hypertrophy of the mandibular elevator muscles.

- Serial cephalometric radiographs offer the most accurate way to determine whether growth has stopped or is continuing.
- The forward positioning of the mandible in a skeletal Class II relationship to make the occlusion look better is known as **Sunday bite.**
- Steep mandibular plane angle correlates with long anterior facial vertical dimensions and anterior bite open bite malocclusion.
- Flat mandibular plane angle correlates with short anterior facial height and deep bite molocclusion.
- **Holdaway ratio** is the relationship between the prominence of the chin (pogonion) compared with the prominence of the lower incisor. The more prominent the chin, the more the lower incisor can be, and vice versa.
- In Ackermann-Profitt classification of malocclusion, the outer envelop describes intra-arch alignment. ***(PGI '06)***
- Timing of orthodontic treatment is during early adolescence, beginning in the late mixed dentition or early adolescence, beginning in the late mixed dentition or early permanent dentition and lasting about 24 months.
- If the second molar has drifted mesially in the space of extracted first molar, it is treated by uprighting the second molar by tipping its crown distally and opening up space for a pontic replacing the missing first molar.
- **Visual Treatment Objectives (VTO)** is a cephalometric tracing representing the changes that are expected during treatment.

- Physiologic response to heavy pressure against a tooth:

Time (seconds)	*Event*
< 1	Periodontal ligament (PDL) fluid in-compressible, alveolar bone bends, piezoelectric signal generated
1-2	PDL fluid expressed, tooth moves within PDL space, no pain
3-5	PDL fluid squeezed out, tissues compressed, immediate pain if pressure is heavy

Optimum forces for orthodontic tooth movement

Type of movement	*Force (gm)*
Tipping	35-60
Bodily movement (translation)	70-120
Root uprighting	50-100
Rotation	35-60
Extrusion	35-60
Intrusion	10-20

- Tipping is the simplest form of orthodontic movement.
- Both continuous and interrupted forces can be produced by fixed appliances that are constantly present.
- Intermittent forces are produced by all patient-activated appliances, such as removable plates, headgear, and elastics. Forces generated during normal function (chewing, swallowing, etc.) can be viewed as a special case of intermittently applied forces.
- Optimum orthodontic tooth movement is produced by **light, continuous force**.
- NiTi alloys have properties of shape memory and super elasticity.
- Elgiloy, the cobalt-chromium alloy has the advantage of formability and can be hardened by heat treatment.

- TMA (Beta-titanium) has desirable combination of strength and springiness (i.e. excellent resilience and good formability).
- The use of rectangular arch wires in rectangular bracket slots was introduced by Edward Angle. The original bracket slot size was 22 × 28 mil (1 mil = 0.01 inch).
- The most commonly missing permanent teeth are the mandibular second premolars and the maxillary lateral incisors.
- Extrusion is the tooth movement that occurs most readily and intrusion occurs least readily.
- 63% of brain case growth is completed at birth. By 15 years, 98% is completed.
- The growth of coronoid process is under the influence of temporalis muscle.
- By two and a half years of age the deciduous dentition is usually complete and in full function.
- The mature swallow are readily observable by 18 months of age.

Facial type	*Dental arch form*
Brachycephalic	Broad
Dolichocephalic	Long and narrow
Mesocephalic	Paraboloid or average

- The term "closed bite" or "deep bite" is a condition of excessive overbite, where the vertical measurement between the maxillary and mandibular incisal margins is excessive when the mandible is brought into habitual or centric occlusion.
- Anteversion **indicates** teeth or other maxillary structures too far forward.

- Intraversion **indicates** teeth or other maxillary structures which are too near from the median plane.
- Supraversion **indicates** teeth or other maxillary structures above their normal vertical relationships.
- Trident of habit factors are duration, frequency and intensity.

Age	*Incidence of diastema*
6	97%
6-7	88%
10-11	48%
12-18	7%

So incidence of diastema is highest at the age of 6 years.

- Ankylosis or partial ankylosis is encountered relatively frequently during the 6 to 12 years age period.
- Essential diagnostic criteria are:
  1. Case history.
  2. Clinical examination.
  3. Plaster study casts.
  4. Radiographs—periapical, bite wing and panoramic.
  5. Facial photographs.
- Supplemental Diagnostic criteria:
  1. a. Cephalometric radiographs.
     b. Occlusal intraoral films.
     c. Selected lateral jaw films.
  2. Electromyographic examination.
  3. Wrist X-rays.
  4. Basal metabolic rate and other endocrine tests.
- **Broadbent registration point** is the midpoint of the perpendicular from the center of sella turcica to the Bolton Plane.

- Angular criteria are the most used of cephalometric analyses. They help in comparing qualitative similarity or difference within the total facial pattern.
- The 45 degree lateral jaw projection gives a more accurate recording of actual tooth positon in either the left or right buccal segment. These projections are of value in following the progress of serial extraction cases and third molar eruption.
- Effects of malocclusions on speech:
  1. An anterior open bite interferes with the normal production of sibilants.
  2. Class II, Division 1 malocclusion with a protruding premaxillary segment makes the normal production of bilabial consonants difficult.
  3. Class III malocclusion, mandibular prognathism, abnormally low tongue position and lethargic tongue function reduce the quality of sibilants.
- Class II malocclusion I has the greatest likelihood of damage to the maxillary incisors as a result of their protruded and relatively unprotected status.
- Edward H. Angle called the first molar the key to occlusion.
- **Denholz appliance** uses muscle anchorage to distally drive first permanent molars.
- The most effective and simplest means of correcting the lingual cross-bite of a maxillary incisor is the use of an acrylic or cast metal inclined plane that is cemented to the mandibular incisors opposing the tooth in cross bite. If properly constructed, it can correct a cross bite in a matter of days.
- Mayne give the mechanisms of incisor liability adjustment:

1. Intercanine arch growth – 3 to 4 mm.
2. Interdental spacing – 2 to 3 mm.
3. More anterior position of permanent incisors as they erupt – 1 to 2 mm.

REMOVABLE AND FIXED APPLIANCES

- Twin-wire attachment was introduced by Joseph Johnson.
- **Baker anchorage** is a type of intermaxillary anchorage.
- **Alveolar bone** has been referred to as **"the slave of the orthodontist"**.
- The Brader arch form for preformed arch wires is based on a trifocal ellipse, which slightly rounds the arch in the premolar region compared with a catenary curve and constricts it posteriorly.
- The safest way to remove metal brackets is to distort the bracket base, which induces failure between it and the bonding adhesive.
- Bonding of bracket is based on the mechanical locking of an adhesive to irregularities in the enamel surface of the tooth and to mechanical locks formed in the base of the orthodontic treatment.
- Straight wire appliance is introduced by Andrews.
- Appliance prescription is the angulation and torque values built into the bracket.
- Removable appliances are indicated primarily for:
  1. Growth modification during the mixed dentition.
  2. Limited (tipping) tooth movements, especially for arch expansion or correction of individual tooth malposition.
  3. Retention after comprehensive treatment.

- Twin block appliance is popularized by Clark and is a modification of the Schwartz double plate mechanism.
- Most screws open 1 mm per complete revolufion, so that a single quarter turn produces 0.25 mm of tooth movement.
- The rate of active movement should not exceed 1 mm per month.
- Expanding the mandibular intercanine distance with an anteriorly positioned screw in a removable appliance is not recommended because the force is concentrated against the incisor and canine teeth so that excessive forces easily can be produced, and because mandibular intercanine expansion is unstable.
- The most useful and versatile clasp for contemporary removable appliances is the Adams Clasp (Crib).
- Labial bow is constructed using 0.7 mm hard round stainless steel wire.
- Force generated by spring is given by

  $$F \times \frac{D^4}{L^3}$$

  where. F = force, D = diameter of wire

  L = length of wire
- Thickness of base plates is 1.5-2 mm. It **offers** adequate strength and tolerated well by patients.
- **Banding** is preferred over bonding in case of posterior teeth.
- Ceramic brackets are made of aluminium oxide or zirconium oxide.
- Lock pins are made of brass.
- **Austenitic stainless steel** is used to make orthodontic arch wires.
- Lingual orthodontic technique was introduced by Craven Kurz.

- Vestibular or oral screen was introduced by Newell.
- Function Regulator appliance was developed by Professor Rolf Frankel.
- Bionator was developed by Balters.
- Indications of Bionator are:
  1. Class II Division I malocclusion with retruded mandible, with labial tipping of upper incisors.
  2. Class III malocclusion.
  3. Open bite.
- The angle between upper and lower bite blocks in Twin block appliance is 45°.
- Herbst appliance, Jasper Jumper, Pendulum appliance are fixed functional appliances. ***(AIPG '04, BHU '06)***
- Herbst appliance is indicated in correction of Class II malocclusions due to retrognathic mandible.
- Jasper Jumper is indicated in skeletal Class II malocclusion with maxillary excess and mandibular deficiency.
- The two blocks in twin block functional appliance are angulated at 70° to the occlusal plane, although the it may be reduced to 45°, if the patient fails to bite forward and thus occlude the blocks. ***(AIPG '04)***
- Head gears are the most commonly used extra oral orthopaedic appliances. They are used to distalize the maxillary dentition or maxilla itself.
- Face mask is used in a growing patient having a prognathic mandible and retrusive maxilla.
- Chin cup is used to restrict the forward and downward growth of the mandible.
- **Hickham** was the first to use face mask or reverse head gear. But Delaire popularized it.

CEPHALOMETRICS

- The distance between the x-ray source and the mid-sagittal plane of the patient is fixed at 5 feet (152.4 cm).
- Bottom point is the highest point at the post condylar notch of the occipital bone.
- Prosthion of supradentale is the lowest and most anterior point on the alveolar bone in the midline, between the upper central incisors.
- Chelion is the lateral terminus of the oral slit on the outer corner of the mouth.
- Sella Nasion plane represents the anterior cranial base.
- Bolton's plane connects the Bolton's points posterior to the occipital condyles and nasion.
- Mandibular plane used in Steiner's analysis is a line connecting gonion and gnathion.
- Down Analysis is based on 20 Caucasian individuals of 12-17 years age group belonging to both the sexes.
- The normal facial angle is 87.8°. ***(BHU '06)***
- The mean value of growth axis Y-axis is 59°.
- An increase of A.N.B. angle more than 2° is indicative of Class II skeletal tendency.
- S. line is a line extending from soft tissue contour of the chin to the middle of an 'S' formed by the lower border of the nose. If the lips are located beyond this line, patient will have convex profile.
- Tweed analysis is used in determining the position of the lower incisor and evaluation of prognosis.

ADDITIONAL HIGH YIELD FACTS

- The spheno-occipital synchondrosis is considered to be the most important growth site of the cranial base. It **becomes** fused in the midline area by 20 years of age.
- Inter-sphenoidal synchondrosis is believed to ossify at birth.
- Among the facial bones, the mandible undergoes the larges amount of growth post-natally and also exhibits the largest variability in morphology.
- The condylar growth rate reaches peak between 12½-14 years. The growth ceases around 20 years of age.
- The neonate is without teeth for about 6 months of life.
- Natal and neonatal teeth show a **familial tendency**.
- The incisal liability is about 7 mm in the maxillary arch and about 5 mm in the mandibular arch.
- The amount of leeway space is about 1.8 mm in the maxillary arch and about 3.4 mm in the mandibular arch.
- Broadbent described the "ugly duckling stage".
- If the curve of spee is extended, it would form a circle of about 4 inch diameter.
- Andrews six keys to normal occlusion are:
  - i. Molar inter-arch relationship.
  - ii. Mesio-distal crown angulation. ***(PGI '06)***
  - iii. Labio-lingual crown inclination.
  - iv. Absence of rotation.
  - v. Tight contacts.
  - vi. Curve of spe.

- The normal curve of spee should not exceed 1.5 mm.
- In Class II subdivision, a Class III molar relation exists on one side and a Class I relation on the other side.
- Transversion is transposition of two teeth.
- Torsiversion is rotation of a tooth around its long axis.
- Lischer gave the term Neutrocclusion, Distocclusion, Mesiocclusion:
  Neutrocclusion - Angle's Class I malocclusion
  Distocclusion - Angle's Class II malocclusion
  Mesiocclusion - Angle's Class III malocclusion
- Simon's law of canine states that orbital plane should pass through the distal third of the upper canine.

Simon's plane	*Term used when dental arch is closer to the plane*	*Term used when the arch is farther from the plane*
1. Frankfort horizontal plane	Attraction	Abstraction
2. Orbital plane	Retraction	Protraction
3. Mid-sagittal plane	Contraction	Distraction

- Traits that are influence by the genes are:
  1. Tooth size.
  2. Tooth shape.
  3. Tooth number.
  4. Crowding/Spacing.
  5. Arch dimension.
  6. Overjet.
  7. Frenum.
  8. Inter-arch variations.
- Rubella infections during pregnancy cause the following congenital malformations in the child:
  a. Dental hypoplasia.

b. **E**xtensive caries. (Mnemonic: RED)
c. **R**etarded eruption of teeth.

- Orthodontic treatment is contraindicated in osteoporosis.
- The habit of thumb and digit sucking is normal till age of 3½-4 years.
- Sears and **Wise** proposed that prolonged suckling can lead to thumb sucking.

Funcional Regulators	*Uses*
FR1	Treatment of Class I Class II Div. I malocclusion
FR2	Treatment of Class II Div. 1 and 2
FR3	Treatment of Class III
FR4	Treatment of open bite and bimaxillary protrusion
FR5	Treatment of long face patients having mandibular plane angle and vertical maxillary excess. They incorporate head gear

- Out of these Functional Regulator, FR2 is the most commonly used appliance.
- Tongue plays an important role in bringing relapse of orthodontically treated case of open bite. ***(BHU '06)***
- Handicapping Labio-Lingual Deviation Index was developed by Harry L. Draker.
- The Orthodontic Treatment Priority Index was developed by Grainger R.M.

TPI scores	*Treatment needs*
0-2.5	Low
2.5-4.5	Middle
above 4.5	High

TPI has been used in epidemiological surveys and serves as an instrument for screening.

- An increase of nasolabial angle more than 110° indicates retrognathic maxilla or retroclined maxillary anteriors.
- H.D. Kesling first proposed the diagnostic set up.
- X-rays was discovered in 1895 (by Roentgen).
- Methods used to assess the skeletal maturity using hand-wrist radiographs are:
  1. Atlas method by Grenlich and Pyle.
  2. Bjork, Grave and Brown Method.
  3. Hagg and Taranger Method.
  4. Fishman's Skeletal Maturity Indicators.
- **Seymour** determined the skeletal maturity based on the mineralisation of the lower canine.
- Theories of tooth movement by orthodontic force:
  1. Pressure tension theory by Schwarz.
  2. Blood flow theory by Bien.
  3. Bone bonding piezoelectric theory by Farrar.
- **Lag phase** of tooth movement is characterized by formation of hyalinized tissue.
- Three processes that takes place during bone resorption are decalcification, degradation of matrix and transport of soluble products to the extracellular fluid and blood vascular system.
- Degradation of matrix is brought about by the activity of Cathepsin B-1.
- Centre of resistance in a single rooted tooth lies between one third and one half of the root, apical to the alveolar crest.
- Centre of resistance in a multi-rooted tooth lies between the roots 1-2 mm apical to the furcation.

- Torquing is a reverse tipping characterized by lingual movement of the root.
- Controlled tipping of a tooth occurs when a tooth tips about a center of rotation at its apex.
- Uncontrolled tipping of a tooth occurs when a tooth tips about a center of rotation apical to and very close to the center of resistance.
- The histological section of tooth under orthodontic force representing an avascular area in the periodontal ligament is often referred as hyalinized zone. *(AIPG '06)*
- Ponts analysis determine how much expansion is possible at the premolar and molar regions. ***(BHU '06)***
- Carey's analysis is done on the lower cost while arch perimeter analysis is done on the upper cost.
- The Bolton's analysis helps in determining dispro-portion in size between macillary and mandibular teeth.
- **Bolton ratio** is the ratio between mesiodistal width of maxillary and mandibular teeth. It is considered as the 7th key to normal occlusion. *(AIPG '04, BHU '06)*
- Moyers analysis evaluate the amount of space available in the arch for the erupting permanent canines and premolars.
- **Tanaka-Johnston Analysis:**
  ½ sum of the mesiodistal width of the 4 lower inci-sors plus 10.5 mm = estimated width of mandibular canine and premolar in one quadrant.
  ½ sum of the width of the 4 lower incisors plus 11.0 mm = estimated width of maxillary canine and premolars in one quadrant.

No radiograph is required in this analysis and is said to be most practical.

- Transient malocclusions or self-correcting malocclusions are:
  a. Open bite seen in the gum pads.
  b. Spacing in desiduous dentition.
  c. Deep bite.
  d. Flush terminal plane.
  e. Ugly duckling stage.
- Milwaukee brace used in the treatment of scoliosis causes retardation of mandibular growth.
- **Kjellgren** coined the term serical extraction.
- Proximal stripping to gain space is done when the space required is 0-2.5 mm.
- Pendulum appliance is used for distalization of molars.
- Emerson C. Angell is considered the father of rapid maxillary expansion.
- The sphenoid bone and the zygomatic bone resist mid-palatal suture opening.
- Maxillary occlusal view radiograph and P.A. Cephalogram are used to estimate the amount of maxillary expansion.
- Tooth and tissue borne fixed expansion appliances are Derichsweiler type and Hass type.
- Tooth borne fixed expansion appliances are Isaacson type and Hyrax type (Hygienic Rapid Expander).
- The force generated by rapid maxillary appliance is 10-20 pounds while the force generated by slow expansion appliance is 2-4 pounds.
- Four helices are incorporated in the quad Helix appliance to increase the flexibility and range of action.

- In Wilkinson extraction all the four first permanent molars are extracted between the age of 8½-9½ years.
- Anterior open bite in a young child with good facial proportions usually needs no treatment, because there is a good chance of spontaneous correction.
- Rapid palatal expansion is done with a jackscrew that is activated at 0.5 to 1 mm per day.
- In camouflage treatment, anteroposterior displacement of the teeth relative to their supporting bone is done. Space is gained by extracting first premolars.
- Camouflage treatment is indicated in:
  a. Too old for successful growth modification.
  b. Mild to moderate skeletal Class II or mild skeletal Class III.
  c. Good vertical facial proportions, neither extreme short face (deep bite) nor long face (open bite).
  d. Reasonable good alignment of teeth.
- **Vitamin D administration** and **injection of prostaglandin** in the periodontal ligament enhance the response to orthodontic treatment.
- Based on the duration of application, force is divided into:
  a. *Continuous force:* Force maintained at some appreciable fraction of the original from one patient visit to the next.
     E.g. light wire appliance.
  b. *Interrupted:* Force levels decline to zero between activation.
     E.g.: Force exerted by extra-oral appliance worn only at night.
  c. *Intermittent:* Force levels decline abruptly to zero intermittently.
     E.g.: Removable plates, elastics, headgear.

- Ectopic eruption of maxillary canines leads to:
  1. Impaction of the canine.
  2. Resorption of permanent lateral incisor roots.
- In a child whose permanent canines have not yet erupted, a diastema of 2 mm or less is likely to close spontaneously. A diastema greater than 2 mm is unlikely to close spontaneously.
- Frenectomy before treatment of midline diastema is contraindicated, and a post-treatment frenectomy should be attempted only if there is a continued tendency of the diastema to reopen and unresolved bunching of tissue between the teeth is present.
- The key to successful intrusion is light continuous force directed toward the tooth apex.
- A 12 to 14-year-old boy in the early permanent dentition with a Class II problem, whose skeletal maturity is somewhat behind his stage of dental development, and who has good growth potential, is best treated by using headgear.
- High pull headgear to the upper molars is the treatment of choice if excessive vertical development of the posterior maxilla is the basic problem. This treatment is continued until growth is nearly complete.
- Teeth require essentially full-time retention after comprehensive orthodontic treatment for the first 3 to 4 months after a fixed orthodontic appliance is removed.
- If the teeth were quite irregular initially, retention should be continued for at least 12 months because of the slow response of the gingival fibres but can be reduced to part-time after 3 to 4 months.

- The best retainer for diastema maintenance is a bonded section of flexible wire. The object of the retainer is to hold the teeth while allowing them some ability to move independently during function.
- The rectangular bracket slot permits control of buccolingual axial inclinations. ***(AIIMS '06)***
- The relatively wide bracket helps control undesirable rotations and tipping.
- The bilateral sagittal split osteotomy (BSSO) of the mandibular ramus, performed from an intra-oral approach is the preferred procedure for mandibular advancement.
- The BSSO and TOVRO (transoral vertical oblique ramus osteotomy) are used to move the mandible posteriorly TOVRO requires full-thickness overlapping of the segments.
- Edwards developed circumferential supracrestal fibrotomy.
- Fixed appliances with multilooped archwires are used in correction of crowding.
- Fixed appliances with elastic chains are used in closure of generalized spacing.
- The deep overbite is treated by using anterior bite plane or fixed appliances incorporating anchor bonds or reverse curve of spee.
- Severe Class III malocclusion with maxillary retrusion can be treated by reverse head gear to protract the maxilla.
- Fixed retainers are band and spur retainer, banded canine to canine retainer, bonded lingual retainer.
- Heat and pressure are involved in spot welding.

- The ratio of the anatomic portion to artistic portion in an ideal study model is 3 : 1.
- Butler's field theory states that mammalian dentition can be divided into molar/premolar field, the canine and the incisor fields.

MISCELLANEOUS

1. Late mesial shift is due to closure of "Leeway space". *(AIPG '96)*
2. Type of Malocclusion — Disease of bones

Type of Malocclusion	Disease of bones
Class III malocclusion (Mnemonic – DACleC)	**D**own's syndrome **A**chondroplasia **Clei**docranial dysplasia **C**raniofacial dysostosis
Class II malocclusion (Mnemonic – PiT)	**Pi**erre Robin syndrome **T**reacher-Collins syndrome

3. The lip is supported by relation of lip edge and facial surfaces of teeth.
4. Open bite on cephalogram shows as increased mandibular plane angle. *(AIPG '97)*

- Skeletal anterior open bite during the mixed dentition period is treated by using a vertical pull head gear with chin up.
- Skeletal anterior open bites is treated during growth by using F.R. IV.
- Fixed appliance in conjunction with box elastics is used to treat mild to moderate open bites.
- **Scissors bite** is a form of posterior cross bite where the maxillary posteriors occlude entirely on the buccal aspect of the mandibular posteriors. *(BHU '06)*

- Tongue blade, Catlan's appliance, Z spring, face mask are used to treat anterior cross bite.
- Cross bite elastic, Coffin spring, Quad helix, Rapid maxillary expansion are used in treatment of posterior cross bite.
- Elastics, closed coil spring, M spring are used to treat midline diastema.
- **Pericision** is generally undertaken as an adjunctive retention procedure **after** the correction of rotations.
- Cases that require prolonged or permanent retention are:
  a. Severe rotations.
  b. Midline diastema.
  c. Arch expansion achieved without good occlusion.
  d. Patients with abnormal muscular or tongue habits.
  e. Expanded arches in cleft palate patients.
- Removable retainers are Hawley's appliance, Begg retainer, Clip on retainer, Wrap around retainer, Invisible retainers, Kesling tooth positioner.

5. Facial form:
   a. **M**esoprosopic - nor**m**al face form
   b. Eu**r**yprosopic - b**r**oad and short face form
   c. **L**eptoprosopic - **l**ong and narrow face form
6. Physique or body build classification:
   a. Aesthetic or ectomorphic - tall and thin physique with narrow dental arches
   b. Pletoric or endomorphic - short and obese physique with large square dental arches
   c. Athletic or meso-morphic - normal or average physique with normal sized dental arches

7. Broadbent registration point is the midpoint of the perpenidicular from the center of sella tursica to the Bolton's plane (a plane that connects Bolton's point and nasion). Superimposition in cephalometric studies is done from registration point and this best demonstrates growth of structures farthest from the point. *(AIIMS '06)*
8. The normal percentage of enlargement or magnification considered normal in cepahlogram is 6-7%. *(AIIMS May '06)*
9. Three dimensional classification of malocclusion (viz. anterior-posterior, transverse, vertical planes) was given by Simon.
10. Centre of rotation in translation is at infinity. *(AIPG '04)*
11. Normal facial index is 80-90%. *(AIPG '04)*

$$\text{Facial index} = \frac{\text{Facial height}}{\text{Zygomatic width}} \times 100$$

$$= \frac{\text{Distance between nasion and gnathion}}{\text{Distance between two zygoma points}} \times 100$$

It determines the overall facial form.

Facial index value	*Facial form*
79-83	Euryprosopic
84-88	Mesoprosopic
89-93	Leptoprosopic

12. A distal shoe type of space maintainer is indicated when the primary 2nd molar is lost before the eruption of permanent 1st molar.
    It is contraindicated in:
    a. Patients with heart disease.
    b. Patients with poor oral hygiene.
    c. Hemophilic patients.

13. The most common complication of the buccal coil spring which is used to regain the space between first premolar and first molar is rotation of first premolar. *(AIIMS '06)*

- Approximately 60% of malocclusion occurs due to premature exfoliation of primary teeth.
- Loss of all permanent first molars results in decrease in 50% of masticatory efficiency.
- Key ridge is the lower most point on the contour of the anterior wall of the infratemporaral fossa (zygoma).

  In deciduous dentition – Zygoma corresponds to maxillary second molar.

  In permanent dentition – Zygoma corresponds to mesiobuccal root of maxillary first molar. *(AIPG '97)*
- Synostosis is early closure of a suture.
- In skeletal Class III malocclusion, there is disturbance in pronunciation of labiodental sounds like 'f', 'v' while in Class II division 2 malocclusion, alveolar sounds like 't' and 'd' are distorted while pronouncing it.
- The twin block appliance was developed by William Clark.
- The nature of **force** produced by **elastics** is **continuous.**

CHAPTER FIVE

Pediatric Dentistry

INTRODUCTION

1. In adult dentistry, the approach is 1:1 (Dentist: Patient) whereas in pediatric dentistry, the approach is 1:2, i.e. child and parent.
2. The Pedodontic treatment triangle was put forth by Dr. G.F. Wright. The child is at the apex of the triangle while the parent and the dentist occupy the base.
3. The U.N. Convention on the Rights of a child was adopted on 20th November 1989.
4. In India, Pediatric Dentistry was first started as a speciality in the year 1962.
5. The Indian Society of Pedodontic and Preventive Dentistry was founded in the year 1979.

THEORIES OF CHILD DEVELOPMENT

1. Psychoanalytical theory by Sigmund Freud.
2. Psychosocial theory by Eric Ericson.
3. Cognitive Theory by Jean Piaget.

CHILD MANAGEMENT

1. Tell-Show-Do technique was given by H.K. Addleston.

2. Hand-Over-Mouth technique was given by Dr. Evangelin.
3. Hand-Over-Mouth exercise (Home or aversive conditioning) is not used routinely but as a last resort method, usually with children 3 to 6 years of age who have appropriate communication abilities. ***(PGI '02)***
4. The intelligence quotient (IQ) formula given by Prof. Binet:

$$IQ = \frac{\text{Mental age}}{\text{Chronologic age}} \times 100$$

IQ range	*General classification*	*Percent of population*
140 and up	Very superior	0.5
120-139	Superior	2.5
110-119	High average	14
90-109	Average	60
80-89	Low average	12
70-79	Borderline impaired	7
69 and below	Mentally retarded	4

DEVELOPMENT ANOMALIES OF THE TEETH

1. **Fusion of the teeth:** It represents the union of two independently developing primary or permanent teeth. It is almost always limited to the **anterior teeth** and shows a **familial tendency**.
2. **Gemination:** It represents an attempted division of a single tooth germ by invagination occurring during the proliferatve stage of the growth cycle of the tooth and shows **familial tendency**.
3. **Dens in Dente (Dens Invaginatus):** It is lingual invagination of the enamel. It is most often seen in permanent maxillary lateral incisors.

EARLY EXFOLIATION OF TEETH

1. **Hypophosphatasia:** Premature exfoliation of the antrior primary teeth is due to deficient cementum. The disease is charactrised by **deficient alkaline phosphatase activity** and **increased levels of urinary phosphoethanolamine**.
2. **Cherubism (Familial Fibrous Dysplasia):** Premature exfoliation of teeth is due to loss of support or root resorption. In permanent teeth, it is due to interference in the development of roots.
3. **Acrodynia (Pink disease):** The exposure of young children to minute amounts of mercury is responsible for the disease. It is called pink disease due to desquamation of the soles and palms. Ointments medications are the usual sources of the mercury.
4. **Familial hypophosphatemia** is Vitamin D-Resistant Rickets.
5. **Cyclic neutropenia:** It is an autosomal dominant condition. There is loss of supporting bone around the teeth.
6. **Premature exfoliation or marked mobility** of teeth in childhood or adult has been associated in some cases with other systemic disorders, acatalasia, Chediak-Higashi syndrome, Down's syndrome, Ehlers-Danlos syndrome, hyperthyroidism, hypertpituitarism, Papillon—Lefevre syndrome.

CAUSES OF ENAMEL HYPOPLASIA

1. Nutritional deficiencies of vitamins A, C and D, calcium and phosphorous.
2. Nephrotic syndrome.

3. Congenital allergies.
4. Lead poisoning (Plumbism).
5. Local infection and trauma.
6. Cleft lip and palate.
7. X-ray radiation and chemotherapy.
8. Rubella embryopathy.

CAUSES OF INTRINSIC DISCOLORATION OF TEETH

1. Hyperbilirubinemia in erythroblastosis fetalis and biliary atresia, premature birth, ABO incompatibility, neonatal respiratory distress, significant internal haemorrhage, biliary hypoplasia, α_1-antitrypsin deficiency, tyrosinemia, neonatal hepatitis, congenital hypothyroidism.
2. Porphyria.
3. Cystic fibrosis.
4. **Tetracycline therapy:** The sensitive period for tetracycline induced discoloration in the permanent maxillary and mandibular incisors and canines is 3 to 5 months postpartum to about the seventh year of the child's life. The maxillary lateral incisors are an exception because they begin to calcify at 10 to 12 months postpartum.

CAUSES OF MACROGLOSSIA

1. Type 2 glycogen storage disease.
2. Neurofibromatosis type 1.
3. Beckwith—Wiedemann syndrome.
4. Down's syndrome.

5. Acromegaly.
6. Cretinism.
7. Myxedema.
   Mnemonic: National Book Trust, Delhi; Master of Computer Application

ANOMALIES OF THE TONGUE

1. Geographic tongue—red, smooth areas devoid of filiform papillae appear on the dorsum of the tongue.
2. White Strawberry tongue—enlargement of the fungiform papillae, observed in cases of scarlet fever and Kawasaki disease.
3. Black hairy tongue—accumulations of Keratin on the filiform papillae become elongated into hairlike processes as long as 1 inch.
4. Crenation—indentation of the tongue margin and is related to pressure habits, macroglossia, and vitamin B-complex deficiency.
5. Median rhomboid glossits—oval, rhomboid shaped reddish patch on the dorsal surface of the tongue anterior to circumvallate papillae. It has no filiform papillae.

DENTAL CARIES

1. Theories of caries development:
   a. Acidogenic theory or Chemico-Parasitic Theory by W.D. Miller.
   b. Proteolysis Theory by Gottlieb.
   c. Proteolysis Chelation Theory by Schatz and Martin.
   d. Autoimmune theory by Jackson.

2. Streptococcus mutans is one of the major and most virulent of the caries producing organisms.
3. Demineralization of tooth starts at pH of 5.5 to 5.2.
4. The greatest amount of demineralization occurs 10 to 15 mm beneath the enamel surface because the outer surface of enamel is far more resistant to demineralization by acid than is the deeper portion of enamel.
5. Massler gave definition of rampant caries.
6. Xylitol is a low-calorie sweetener that inhibits the growth of Streptococcus mutans.
7. The route of administration of caries vaccine is mucosal absorption by intraoral or intranasal tissues.
8. The **Vipeholm study** was conducted by Gustaffson *et al.* It showed that the physical form of carbohydrates (stickiness, oral clearance time, frequency of intake) was much more important in cariogenicity than was the total amount of sugar ingested.

Classification of sugar substitutes

Non-caloric sweeteners	**Caloric sweeteners**
1. Aspartame	1. Glycitols
2. Cyclamate	2. Sorbitol
3. Saccharine	3. Xylitol
	4. Mannitol
	5. Lactitol

9. Detection of caries:
   a. Infrared Laser Fluorescence (Diagnodunt).
   b. Digital Imaging **Fiber**-Optic Trans-Illumination.
   c. Quantitative light fluorescence.

d. Electrical conductance measurement.
e. Xeroradiography.

10. Caries Activity Tests:
    a. Lactobacillus colony count test by Hadley.
    b. Snyder test.
    c. Alban test (simplified substitute for Snyder test).
    d. Reductase test (Susceptibility test).
    e. Buffer capacity test.
    f. Swab test by Grainger.

11. Composition of media used for Snyder and Alban test:

Bactopeptone	=	20 grams
Dextrose	=	20 grams
Nacl	=	5 grams
Agar	=	16 grams
Bromocresol green	=	0.02 grams

12. Indication from counts of lactobacilli/ml of saliva lactobacillus colony count test:

No of colony per c.c.	**Degree of caries activity**
0–1000	Little or none
10^3–5000	Slight
5000–10^4	Medium
> 10^4	High

13. Snyder test:

Caries	*Colour change from blue-green to yellow*
High	24 hours
Medium	48 hours
Slight	72 hours
Immune	No change > 72 hours

14. In India dental caries prevalence is higher in urban as compared to rural areas.

ERUPTION OF THE TEETH

1. Sequence of calcification of primary teeth is central incisor, first molar, lateral incisor, canine and second molar.
2. Tooth eruption is influenced by pituitary growth hormone and thyroid hormone.
3. The interval from crown completion and the beginning of eruption until the tooth is in full occlusion is approximately 5 years for permanent teeth.
4. The eruption of primary teeth is preceded by increased salivation, and the child wants to put the hand fingers into the mouth.
5. Eruption sequestrum is seen occasionally in children at the time of eruption of first permanent molar.
6. 85% of natal or neonatal teeth are mandibular primary incisors and few are supernumerary teeth.

Difference among epstein pearls, bohn nodules and dental lamina cysts

Epstein pearls	*Bohn modules*	*Dental lamina cysts*
1. Form along the mid-palatine raphe	1. Form along the buccal and lingual aspects of dental ridges and on the palate away from the raphe	1. Form on the crest of the maxillary and mandibular ridge
2. Remnants of epithelial tissue trapped along the raphe	2. Remnants of mucous gland tissue	2. Remnants of dental lamina

CAUSES OF DELAYED ERUPTION OF TEETH

1. Ankylosed teeth.
2. Down syndrome.

3. Cleidocranial Dysplasia (Mutational dysostosis, cleidocranial dysostosis, Marie-sainton syndrome).
4. Hypothroidism.
5. Hypopituitarism.
6. Achondroplastic dwarfism.
7. Fibromatosis gingivae.
8. Gardner syndrome.
9. Hunter syndrome.
10. Progeria syndrome.
11. Familial Hypophosphatemia.

- For children tooth brush with soft bristle, smaller head, thicker handle and shorter bristle length than adult-size brush is advised.
- Unwaxed nylon filament floss is the floss of choice due to ease of **passing** the floss between tight contacts, lack of wax residue, the squeaking sound effect produced by moving the floss over a clean tooth, and the fiber spread which results in increased surface contact and greater plague removal.
- Disclosing agents of plague:

  Iodine, gentian violet, **erythrosin**, basic fuchsin, fluorescein.

GROWTH AND DEVELOPMENT

- Theories of Growth:
  a. Functional matrix theory by Moss.
  b. Sutural theory of growth by Sicher.
  c. Cartilagenous theory of growth.
- The Frankfort horizontal plane is an anthropometric reference line used for analysis of the **lateral** face.
- Enlow demonstrated that the facial profile flattens as the face ages.

- By 3 years of age, the occlusion of 20 deciduous teeth is established.
- Dental size is expressed through X-linked inheritance.
- Crowding is the most common features of dental arch malocclusion.
- Sevoflurane is the general anaesthesia of choice in children because it is associated with less myocardial depression and fewer and less significant respiratory problems when used for inhalational induction.
- Root canal filling material for primary teeth and their composition.
  1. KRI paste—Iodoform, camphor, parachlorophenol, menthol.
  2. Vitapex—Calcium hydroxide, iodoform.
  3. Walkhoff paste—Parachlorophenol, camphor, menthol.
  4. Maisto paste—ZnO, iodoform, **thymol**, camphor, lanolin.
- The main advantages of KRI paste compared with zinc oxide-eugenol paste are that KRI paste resorts in synchrony with primary roots and is less irritating to surrounding tissues.
- **Herman** introduced $Ca(OH)_2$ as a dressing agent for pulp.
- The greatest increase in the incidence of gingivitis in children is seen in the age of 6-7 years. It is because the gingival margin receives no protection from the coronal contour of the tooth during the early stage of active eruption.
- The peak age for recurrent aphthous ulcer is between 10 and 19 years of age.
- The causative gene for papillon-Lefevre Syndrome is located at chromosome band **11q14-q21**.

EXTRINSIC STAINS ON TEETH

1. Green stain is due to the action of chromogenic bacteria on the enamel cuticle, more in mouth breathers.
2. Orange stain is due to poor oral hygience, present in the gingival third of the tooth.
3. Black stain-relatively resistant to caries

- Storage medium for avulsed teeth are:
  1. Milk.
  2. Isotonic saline.
  3. Patient's saliva.

- Children with Down Syndrome are cooperative and dental procedures can be provided if the dentist works at a slightly slower pace.
- The amount of fluoride present in blood is 0.10 to 0.15 ppm and in saliva 0.1 ppm.
- Folic acid (pterylglutamic acid, folacin) plays a role in the synthesis of purine and pyrimidine compounds.
- Pellagra is characterized by large, symmetrically developed patches of erythema on the forearms face, neck, and backs of the hands.
- Calcium, phosphorous, iron absorption are enhanced by acid pH in the intestine.
- **Herpangina (Summer disease)** is caused by Coxsackie A viruses.
- Hand, foot and Mouth Disease is caused by coxsackie A16 virus.
- If a pregnant woman contracts German measles during the first fourteen weeks of pregnancy, the foetus will have some abnormality like cleft palate and others dental anomalies.
- Strawberry tongue is seen in scarlet fever (Scarlatina).
- Prophylactic odontotomy is popularized by Hyatt and *et al.*

- Supernumerary permanent teeth are relatively frequent while supernumerary primary teeth are very rare.
- In formocresol pulpotomy, formocresol creates a zone of fixation, which is bacteria free and inert, resistant to autolysis and acts as a deterrent to further microbial infiltration.
- Pulp capping is the simplest form of pulp therapy.
- The purpose of carving is to conform to the original anatomy of the tooth.
- Research has shown that the force needed to withdraw pins of the friction-locked type may be as high as1600 psi.
- The most generally used intra-oral film is the No. 1.2 in children.
- A film's emulsion speeds is classified as A, B, C, D, E, F. A is the slowest film available and F is the fastest.
- When high contrast is needed, to detect small carious lesions, the lower KvP are used (KvP varies from 60 to 100).
- When the tube to film distance is increased by double, the exposure time must be multiplied by four.
- The greater the milliamperage is, the less exposure time needed.
- Deep bites are most often observed in class II, Division I malocclusion.
- **Baume** gave the term 'primate space'.
- Mandibular third molars are the most frequently impacted teeth. Maxillary permanent canines are the next.
- The primary purpose of completing palate by 2 years of age is to facilitate the acquisition of normal speech.

Site of insertion of needle for inferior alveolar nerve block in children:		
< 6 years	:	below occlusal plane
6-12 years	:	at occlusal plane
> 12 years	:	above occlusal plane

- A child-visiting dentist for the first time has basic fear of **unknown**.
- The basic fear of a child below 2 years on his first dental visit is fear of being separated from parents. ***(AIPG '91)***
- A 4-year-old child who is aggressive in dental office is due to fear.
- **Transillumination** of soft tissue is useful in detection of Sialolithiasis. ***(AIIMS '94)***
- The first step in treating rampant caries is excavation of softened tooth structure and filling with zinc oxide eugenol. ***(PGI '96)***
- Adequate local anesthesia for upper primary second molar can be secured by buccal and palatal infiltration. ***(AIPG '97)***
- Paradoxical excitation in children is caused by barbiturates. Hence, it is contraindicated in children. ***(PGI '01, BHU '06)***
- Claustrophobia is fear of closed spaces like "Dental clinics".
- 20-40% N_2O used in conscious sedation causes floating sensation euphoric state (laughing sensation).
- Incidence of caries is less in patients with Down's Syndrome.

- The source of calcium ions of a calcific bridge in a tooth in which calcium hydroxide pulpotomy has been done is blood vessel borne. ***(AIIMS '99)***
- Exarticulation of teeth means avulsion. ***(PGI '02)***
- Partial pulpotomy technique was advocated by **Cvek.** ***(AIPG '06)***
- Distal shoe was first advocated by Willet. ***(AIPG'06)***
- Parrot like repetitive speech is found in Autism. ***(PGI '97)***
- Treatment of severe intraoral infections in children differs from that in adult because dehydration occurs more rapidly and severely in children. ***(AIPG '92, BHU '06)***
- Patients with Down's Syndrome normally have Brachycephalic skull. ***(AIPG '04)***
- Granular cell myoblastoma shows epithelial pseudoepithelio-matous hyperplasia. ***(AIIMS 2000)***
- At birth child shows marked convex profile. This is due to small sized mandible. ***(AIIMS '03)***
- Fusion of mandibular symphysis occurs at 18 months. ***(AIIMS '94)***
- Stainless steel crown is developed by Humphrey. ***(AIIMS '06)***
- Psychological basis of 'Tell-show-do' technique is de-sensitization due to familiarity.
- Best approach for managing a 6-year-old child with tamper tantrum is voice control.
- Peer group identity is strongest at teenager. ***(AIPG '03)***

- Dental caries in primary dentition is highest at age group of 2-3 years.
- Breastfeeding should stop at 1½ years of age.
- In a **spaced** primary dentition with a straight terminal plane a class I permanent molar relationship is achieved by **early mesial shift**.
- The **congenital absence** of lateral incisor is attributed to a defect in **initiation** stage of tooth development.
- Chloral hydrate is widely used for pediatric patients.
- Strawberry tongue is associated with scarlet fever. The peak incidence of scarlet fever occurs in children of 4 to 8 years old.
- An outstanding oral manifestation of both ectodermal dysplasia and cleidocranial dysplasia is retained primary teeth.
- **Hemangioma** is the most common benign tumour of infants.
- Overcrowding of teeth is present in achondroplasia.
- Acute lymphocytic leukemia is the most common cancer found in pediatric patients.
- Porphyria patients has the following symptoms:
  1. Red urine.
  2. Purplish-brown teeth.
  3. Sensitivity to sunlight.
  4. Blisters with swelling on the face hands when exposed to sunlight (photodermatitis).
  5. Visceral complaints (abdominal pain, cramping etc.).
  6. Neuropsychiatric complaints.
- Gingivostomatitis is common, particularly among **children**.

CHAPTER SIX

Complete Denture

- The epithelium tlat lines the oral cavity is the stratified squamous.
- On the ventral surface of the caviar tongue, there is nodular varicose enlargement of the veins. It is commonly seen in the elderly edentulous patient.
- Dr. Robert Moyers first used electromyography in dentistry.
- The basic structural change in reduction of residual ridges is a reduction in the size of the bony ridge under the mueoperiosteum.
- **De Van** gave the neutrocentric concept of using flat teeth.
- For denture construction process, serous type of saliva is the best to work with.
- The U-shaped palatal vault is most favourable for retention and lateral stability.
- Papillary hyperplasia is caused by local irritation, poor oral hygiene, and low-grade infections such as Monilia.
- Epulis fissuratum results from chronic irritation of a poorly fitting denture flange on the **sulcular** epithelium.

- The ideal shape of the maxillary edentulous ridge is the U-shape with parallel walls and a broad, well-rounded crest.
- Tori are composed of laminated cortical bone covered with a thin layer of mucosa.
- Mandibular tori or torus mandibularis occur commonly on the medial surface of the mandible in the canine premolar region bilaterally.
- Composition of tissue conditioners:
  1. Polyethyl methacrylate.
  2. Aromatic ester ethyl alcohol mixture.

  The main reason for the use of tissue conditioners is to aid or prevent in the treatment of chronic soreness from dentures.
- Tissue conditioners roughen and harden within four to eight weeks.
- Distolateral termination of the maxillary denture base lies in the hamular notch.
- Mean denture bearing area of edentulous maxilla is 22.96 cm^2 and 12.25 cm^2 in an edentulous mandible.
- Area of periodontal ligament available in each of the arch (maxilla or mandible) is 45cm^2.
- Morphologic changes associated with the edentulous condition are:
  1. **Deep**ening of nasolabila groove.
  2. **D**ecrease in horizontal labial angle.
  3. **N**arrowing of lips. *(AIPG '04)*
  4. **I**ncrease in columella-philtsal angle.
  5. **Pro**gnathic appearance.
  6. **L**oss of labiodental angle.

  Mnemonic: **Pro Deep INDia Limited.**

- Papillary hyperplasia is associated with wearing of dentures with relief chambers.
- Palatal papillomatosis is related to wearing of maxillary denture with a suction cup.
- Denture sore mouth is due to underlying abnormal metabolic or hormonal function or a nutritional deficiency. ***(PGI '92)***
- The most important diagnostic information to be obtained from mounted diagnostic casts is related to the occlusion.
- The chewing efficiency of the average denture wearer is about 20% that of an adult with complete natural dentition.
- The objectives of an impression are to provide:
  1. Retention.
  2. Stability.
  3. Support.
- Retention for denture is the resistance to removal in direction opposite that of its insertion.
- Stability for denture is the quality of beings firm, steady and constant in position when horizontal forces are applied to it.
- Support is the resistance of denture to the vertical components of mastication and to occlusal or other forces applied in direction toward the basal seat.
- Factors of retention of dentures:
  1. Adhesion.
  2. Cohesion.
  3. Interfacial surface tension.
  4. Capillary attraction.

5. Atmospheric pressure.
6. Oral and facial musculature.

- **Atmospheric pressure** is an emergency retentive force.
- The area between the mandibular buccal frenum and the anterior edge of the masseter is known as the buccal shelf. Buccal shelf is the main stress bearing area of the mandible.
- The distal end of the lingual flange of mandibular denture is limited by the glossopalatine arch, which is formed by the glossopalatine muscle and the lingual extension of the superior constrictor muscle. ***(AIPG '04, BHU '06)***
- The crest of the lower residual ridge is not favourable as the primary stress-bearing area for a lower denture because the underlying bone is cancellous.
- **Christiansen phenomenon** are the concurrent changes seen in the vertical dimensions between the posterior upper and lower residual alveolar ridges when the articulating eminences push the mandibular condyles downward as the mandible is moved forward or laterally.
- The condyle can translate 18 mm (3/4 inch) approximately. ***(PGI '99)***
- Bennet shift is the direct lateral side shift of the mandible that occurs simultaneously with a lateral excursion. It is due to mesial (inward) movement of the balancing condyle with a corresponding lateral (outward) movement of the working conyle.
- Chewing **center** is located within the brain stem (specifically in the reticular formation of the pons).

- The vertical jaw relations are established by the mandibular musculature in infants and edentulous adults.
- Mechanical methods of determining the vertical dimension are:
  1. Ridge relation.
  2. Measument of the former dentures.
  3. Preextraction records.
- Physiologic methods or determining the vertical dimension are:
  1. Physiologic rest position.
  2. Phonetics and esthetics.
  3. Swallowing threshold.
  4. Patient-reported perception of comfort.
  5. Jactile sense.
- The stability of the denture bases is disturbed and there is unnecessary pain or discomfort in the edentulous patient when the centric relation and centric occlusion do not coincide in artificial teeth or a freedom in centric is not present.
- **Hanau** referred to tissue resiliency as realeff, an acronym for phase **re**silienc**y** **a**nd **l**ike **eff**ect. This resiliency in present in both the **TMJs** or mucosa.
- Fish described a dentures as having three surfaces: the impression, the occlusal and the polished surface.
- **The modiolus** is formed by the meeting of orbicularis oris, triangularis, buccinator, risorius, zygomaticus major, caninus, quadratus labii superioris, quadratus labii inferioris.

Width of the upper central incisor is approximately 1/16 bizygomatic width.

Width of the upper six anterior teeth is 1/33 the bizygomatic width.

- The dentogenic concept in selecting artificial teeth is based on the age, sex and personality of the patient.
- Teeth with 30-degree cuspal inclinations are the most effective for checking the accuracy of jaw relations.
- Three specifications for teeth in centric occlusion:
  1. The upper should overlap the lower teeth.
  2. The long axis of each upper tooth should be distal to the long axis of the corresponding lower tooth.
  3. Each tooth except the lower central incisor and the upper last molar should be opposed by two teeth.
- The dentist has no control over patients condylar inclination but the incisal guide angle is established by the dentist within the limits of esthetics.
- Hanau stated the five principal factors in the laws of occlusion for protrusive movement:
  1. Inclination of the condylar guidance.
  2. Inclination of the incisal guidance.
  3. Orientation of the occlusal plane.
  4. Inclination of the cusp.
  5. Prominence of the compensating curve.
- The average Bennett shift is 15°.
- The minimum level for implant success is 85% at the end of a 5-year observation period and of 80% at the end of a 10 year period. ***(AIPG '04)***
- The retromolar pad must be covered by the denture base. It aids in the stability of the denture by adding another plane to resist movement of the base.
- Retromolas pad contains:
  1. Fibers of the pterygomandibular raphe.

2. Fibers of the superior pharyngeal constrictor.
3. Fibers of the buccinator muscles.
4. Fibers of the temporal tendon and glandular tissue.

- The mylohyboid muscle influences the mid and anterior portions of the inferior border of the lingual flange.
- Functional movements of the stomatognathic system are mastication, deglutition and phonation.
- The primary purpose of the posterior palatal seal is the retention of the maxillary denture.
- The correctly placed posterior palatal seal create a partial vacuum beneath the maxillary denture. This partial vacuum is activated only when horizontal or tipping forces are directed against the denture base.
- Mouth temperature waxes which are used for the location and transfer marking of the anterior and posterior vibrating lines by fluid wax technique are:
  1. Iowa wax—white- by Earl S. Smith.
  2. H-L physiologic paste—yellow-white—by C.S. Harkins.
  3. Adaptol-green—by Nathan O. Kaye.
  4. Koreeta Wax No. 4—orange—O.C. Applegate.
- The maximum depression (downward and forward position) of the soft palate is recorded when the Frankfort plane is 30° below the horizontal and the tongue is firmly positioned against the mandibular anterior teeth.
- The most common cause for failure of the seal in the posterior palatal area is the underextended distal denture border.
- The pterygoid hamuli should not be covered by the denture base because if covered, patient will feel sharp pain during function.

- The posterior palatal seal area lies between the anterior and posterior vibrating lines. The anterior vibrating line is an imaginary line located at the junction of the attached tissues overlying the hard palate and the movable tissues of the immediately adjacent soft palate. The posterior vibrating line is located at the junction of soft palate that has limited or shallow movement during function and the remainder of the soft palate that is markedly displaced during functional movements.
- The posterior vibrating line marks the most distal extension of the denture base. It is an imaginary line located at the junction of the aponeurosis of the tensor veli palatini muscle and the muscular portion of the soft palate.
- While setting posterior teeth, the posterior plane of occlusion should be at a level between 1/3 to 2/3 the height of the retromolar pad.
- Muyskems says, "For every 1 mm the incisal edges of the mandibular anterior teeth are posterior to their normal arrangement, the tongue is deprived of approximately 100 cubic mm of space in which to function".
- **Leon Williams** gave the theory of matching teeth to face forms, which have generally square, tapering or ovoid characteristics.
- Hall introduced inverted cusp.
- The primary function of compensating curve is to provide balancing occlusal contacts for protrusive mandibular positions.
- The main purpose of try-in of denture is to compare the general tooth and arch position with the way the teeth might have grown.

- The forces used during trial closures and final closures of flask are 1500 psi and 3500 psi respectively. *(BHU '06)*
- Denture look or collapsed appearance in complete dentures is due to constricted arch form.
- The most common denture fractures are those along the mandibular and maxillary midline.
- The most important advantage of immediate complete denture is that at no time patient will be without teeth. So, they are able to continue their social and business activities without embarrassment.
- Interim dentures are advised for patients with severe periodontal diseases. There will be preservation of the maximum amount of ridge bulk with the minimum of trauma and swelling.
- Advantages of an overdenture are:
  1. Preservation of alveolar bone.
  2. Support.
  3. Retention.
  4. Periodontal maintenance.
- The primary function of the articulator is to simulate the patient's temporomandibular joints, muscles of mastication, mandibular ligaments, mandible and maxilla, and the complex neuromuscular mechanism that programs mandibular movements.
- Slab articulators were the first articulator.

Class I articulator	Class II A articulator	Class II B articulator
1. Hinge-joint articulator	1. Grittman articulator	1. Monsoon maxillo-mandular articulator
2. Barn-door hinge articulator	2. Gysi simplex articulator	

Class II C articulator

1. The house articulator

Class III A articulator	Class III B articulator
1. Hanau Model H	1. Gysi Trubyte
2. Dentatus	2. Hanau Kinoscope
3. Bergstrom Arcon	3. Stansberry Tripod
	4. Ney
	5. Hanau university series 130-21
	6. Teledyne
	7. Panadent

Class IV A articulator	Class IV B articulator
1. TMT articulator	1. Stuart
	2. Denar D4A
	3. Denar D5A
	4. Simulator.

- The term arcon is used to indicate an instrument that has its condyles on the lower member and the condylar guides on the upper member.

Arcon articulator	Non-arcon articulator
1. Bergstrom Arcon	1. Gysic-Trubyte
2. Ney	2. Hanau Model H
3. Teledyne	3. Dentatus
4. Panadent	
5. Whip-Mix	
6. Omni	
7. Hanau Mate	
8. Denar	

- The Pantronic is an electronic pantograph which provides a computer print-out of numerical condylar measurements.

- Hanau's equation:

$$L = \frac{H}{8} + 12, \text{ where}$$

H = horizontal condylar inclination,
L = Bennettt angle

- In Hanau H2 articulator, the intercondylar distance is fixed at 110 mm.
- In whip-mix articulator, the intercondylar distance is adjustable to three positions: small (S), 96 mm; medium (M), 110 mm; and large (L), 124 mm.
- Face-bow used to record the relationship of the jaws to the temporomandibular joints and to orient casts in the same relationship to the opening axis of the articulator.
- The fork of arbitrary face-bow is attached to the maxillary occlusion rim while the fork of kinematic face-bows is attached to the mandibular occlusion rim.
- Phonetics and anterior teeth:

Sounds	*Letters/words*
1. Labial sounds	b, p, m
2. Labio dental sounds	f, v
3. Dental sounds	'th'in this, that, these, those
4. Alveolar sounds	t, d, n, s, z
5 Palatal sounds	year, vision, onion
6. Velar sounds (posterior)	k, g, ng
7. Sibilant sounds	s, 3, sh , ch , j
8. Voice sounds	a, e, i, o, u, b, d, g, j, v, m, n, e and r

- Articulators that will accept face bow transfer are class III-A and B, class IV-A and B articulators.

ADDITIONAL HIGH YIELD FACTS

1. Metallic oxide paste is carried in a custom tray. *(AIIMS '98)*

2. Oral tissues are best recorded in functional state by selective minimum pressure technique. *(AIPG '94)*
3. Posterior palatal seal is recorded when the head is bent at 30°. *(AIPG '04)*
4. The coronoid process limits the thickness of the distobuccal flange of the upper complete denture. *(AIPG '02).*
5. Bennett movement of mandible is related to lateral bodily movement of mandible. *(AIPG '94)*
6. Hinge axis is located with help of kinematic face bow. *(AIPG '96)*
7. Most reliable method of recording centric relation is graphic tracing with excursive movements. *(AIIMS '94)*
8. Boucher's method of relining is open mouth technique. *(AIPG 2000)*
9. Functional technique of relining and rebasing utilizes tissue conditioner. *(AIPG '02)*
10. Ear prosthesis and ocular prosthesis is made from silicone. *(BHU '06)*
11. A patient complains of looseness of dentures within two to four hours of insertion. This is due to deflective occlusion. *(AIIMS 2000)*
12. A patient complains of generalized soreness over the entire mandibular ridge. This is probably due to excessive vertical dimension. *(AIPG '99)*
13. Number of swallowings per day is 600. *(PGI '03)*
14. Loosing of denture while smiling is due to inadequate relief of the buccal frenum.
15. The width of the posterior palatal seal area is 1-5 mm.
16. An alginate impression is removed with a quick jerk to prevent permanent deformation. *(BHU '06)*

17. Porosity that occurs in the bulky portions of the heat cure acrylic complete dentures is due to direct placement of the packed resin in water at 100°. *(BHU '06)*
18. The main disadvantage of relining and rebasing the complete dentures is change in **centric relation**.
19. Maxillary anterior teeth will produce pleasing effect when placed facial to the alveolar ridge. *(AIPG '04)*
20. Translatory movements of the condyle and the articular disk are controlled by capsular ligament and the suprachead of the lateral pterygoid.

- Proper lip support to the patient with the complete dentures is provided by the facial surfaces of the anterior teeth and the simulated attached gingiva.
- The most common difficulty associated with patients suffering from neuromuscular disorders in construction of a complete denture is recording jaw relations.
- The distofacial border of the mandibular complete denture is limited by the action of masseter.
- Complete dentures are said to be in 'balanced occlusion' when simultaneous contacts occur bilaterally in all eccentric movements. *(BHU '06)*
- Anatomic teeth used in complete dentures have cuspal inclines of 33°.
- Only pure hinge movements of the mandible occur at terminal hinge position. *(AIPG '06, BHU '06)*
- If anterior teeth contacts are present in centric relation when a upper complete denture versus lower anterior natural teeth, it results in **excessive resorption of the upper anterior ridge** and **epulis fissuratum**. *(BHU '06)*

CHAPTER SEVEN

Removable Partial Denture

- Components of removable partial denture are:
  1. Major connectors.
  2. Minor connectors.
  3. Rests.
  4. Direct retainers.
  5. Indirect retainers.
  6. One or more bases and replacement teeth.
- The basic form of lingual bar is half-pear shape with its greatest bulk at the inferior border.
- When wide diastema exist between the lower anterior teeth, a continuous bar (**cingulum bar**) is used.
- Hinged continuous labial bar is a modification to the linguoplate.
- Swing-lock design consists of a labial or buccal bar that is connected to the major connector by a hinge on one end and a latch at the other end.
- Indications of Swing-Lock concept are:
  1. Missing key abutments.
  2. Unfavourable tooth contours.
  3. Unfavorable soft tissue contours.
  4. Teeth with questionable prognosis.
- Contraindications of Swing-Lock concept are:
  1. Poor oral hygiene.

2. Shallow buccal or labial vestbule.
3. High frenal attachment.

- For using lingual bar as major connector, at least 8 mm of vertical space between the active tissues of the floor of the mouth and the gingival margins of the teeth is required. This makes the lingual bar to have a width or height of 5 mm and an essential space of 3 mm between the gingival margin and the superior border of the bar.
- In a patient with bilateral distal extension edentulous areas with resorption of residual ridges, a lingual plate major connector is used.
- Double lingual bar or Kennedy Bar is lingual plate with metal removed from below superior margin of plate down to half pear shaped bar.
- Labial bar, lingual bar and linguoplate are all half pear shape.
- The U-shaped palatal connector is the least desirable of maxillary major connectors.
- The single palatal bar is the most widely used of all palatal major connectors. It is less than 8 mm in width.
- Blatterfein gave a systematic approach to designing maxillary major connector.
- Complete palatal coverage major connector is the most rigid major connector.
- **Beading** is the scribing of a shallow groove not in excess of 0.5 mm in width or depth on the maxillary master cost outlining the palatal major connector exclusive of rugae areas.
- Purposes of beading are:
  1. Transfer of the major connector design to the investment cast.

2. To provide a visible finishing line for the casting.
3. To ensure intimate tissue contact of the major connector with selected palatal tissues.

- The primary function of minor connectors is to join the major connector or base of a removable partial denture with the other components of the prosthesis, such as the clasp assembly, indirect retainers, occlusal rests, or cingulum rests.
- Minor connectors that join denture base to major connector are:
  1. Lattice work type.
  2. Mesh type.
  3. Bead type (used with metal base).
  4. Wire or nail head type (used with metal base).
- The lattice work minor connector provides the strongest attachment of the acrylic resin denture base to the removable partial denture.
- The mesh type of minor connector consists of a thin sheet of metal with multiple small holes that extends over the crest of the residual ridge to the buccal, lingual and posterior limits.
- The bead, wire or nailhead minor connector is used with metal denture base. The denture base is attached to the outer or superior surface of the metal base and retention is gained by projections of metal in the form of bead, wire, nailhead on this surface.
- There is no relief beneath the bead, wire, or, nailhead minor connector while lattice work and mesh minor connectors have space between them and the underlying ridge.
- **Tissue stops** are made by removing approximately 2 mm^2 of the relief wax so that there is direct contact of

the metal with the alveolar ridge. They provide stability and prevent distortion of the framework during acrylic resin processing procedures.

- Tissue stops should engage both buccal and lingual slopes of the residual ridge for stability.
- The finishing line junction between the major connector and the acrylic resin should not be greater than 90°.
- Approach arm of a vertical projection or bar type clasp is the only minor connector which is not rigid.
- The first tissue reaction to metallic coverage is pressure resulting from lack of support.
- Rests prevent vertical movement of the prosthesis toward the tissue and also help to dissipate horizontal forces.
- The outline form of an occlusal rest should be saucer-shaped or rounded triangular shape or spoon shaped.
- The deepest part of an occlusal rest is inside lowered marginal ridge.
- The angle formed by the occlusal rests and the vertical minor connector should be less 90°.

Form of rests	**Tooth on which they are usually made**
1. Occlusal rests	Posterior tooth
2. Lingual or cingulum rest	Maxillary canine
3. Incisal rests	Mandibular canine

- The occlusal rest should be at least 0.5 mm thick at its thinnest point and should be 1.0 –1.5 mm thick where it crosses the marginal ridge.

- Main advantages of internal occlusal rest:
  1. Facilitates the elimination of visible clasp arm buccally.
  2. Permits the location of the rest seat in a more favourable position in relation to the tipping axis of the abutment.
- The preparation of occlusal rest seats should always follow proximal preparation, never precede it.
- The rest seat for lingual rest is V-shaped.
- A lingual rest is always preferred over an incisal rest because it is closer to center of rotation of tooth or placed nearer the horizontal axis of rotation (tipping axis) of the abutment. Hence less tendency to tip the tooth.
- An incisal rest is more likely to lead to some orthodontic movement of the tooth because of unfavorable leverage factors than is lingual rest.
- An incisal rest seat should be approximately 2.5 mm wide and 1.5 mm deep and is placed at the incisal angles of anterior teeth.
- **The intracoronal retainer** (or internal attachment or precision attachment) was developed by Dr. Herman E.S. Chayes.
- Advantages of internal attachment:
  1. Elimination of visible retentive and support components.
  2. Better vertical support through a rest seat located more favorably in relation to the horizontal axis of the abutment tooth.
- The extracoronal direct retainer (or clasp) functions on the principle of the resistance of metal to defor-

mation. It is this resistance to deformation that generates retention.

- **Cone theory**, the basis for clasp retention was given by **Prothero.**
- The only universally flexible form of the clasp arm is the round form.
- The basic principle of clasp design is that more than 180 degrees of the greatest circumference of the crown of the tooth must be included, passing from diverging axial surfaces to converging axial surfaces.
- Tightening a clasp against the tooth or loosening it away from the tooth surfaces increases or decreases frictional resistance and does not affect the retentive potential of the clasp.
- Adjustments in the retention provided by a cast clasp arm is made by moving a clasp terminal cervically into the angle of cervical convergence or occlusally into a lesser area of undercut.
- The T and Y clasp arms of bar clasp are the most frequently misused clasp arm.
- The bar clasp design is based on RPI system where R is rest (mesio-occlusal rest), P is proximal plate and I is I – bar.
- The combination clasp consists of a wrought-wire retentive clasp arm and a cast reciprocal clasp arm. Flexibility, adjustability and the appearance of the wrought wire retentive arm are the advantages of it.
- Combination clasp is preferred over cast circumferential clasp arm and bar clasp arm for use on terminal abutments when torque and tipping are possible because of engaging an undercut away from the distal extension base.

- Function and position of clasp parts.

Component	Function	Location
1. Rest	Support	Occlusal incisal, lingual
2. Minor connector	Stabilization	Proximal surfaces extending from a prepared marginal ridge to the junction of the middle and gingival one third of the abutment tooth
3 Retentive clasp arm	Retention	Gingival one third or crown
4. Reciprocal clasp arm	Stabilization (reciprocation)	Middle one third of crown

- Retention of a clasp depends on the following factors:
  1. Size of the angle of cervical convergence (depth of undercut).
  2. Amount of placement of the clasp terminal into the angle of cervical convergence.
  3. Flexibility of the clasp arm, which is product – of its length, its relative diameter, its cross-sectional form or shape, the material of which it in made.
- Functions of the reciprocal clasp arm:
  1. It should provide stabilization and reciprocation against the action of the retentive arm.
  2. It should be located so that the denture is stabilized against horizontal movement. Stabilization is achieved by the use of rigid clasp arms, rigid minor connectors, and a rigid major connector.
  3. It acts to a minor degree as an indirect retainer.
- Chrome alloys have higher modulus of elasticity than gold alloys and are therefore less flexible.
- The tensile strength of a wrought structure is at least 25% greater than that of the cast alloy from which it was made.
- Clasp of choice for tipped molars is ring clasp.

- The approach arm of bar clasp should cross the gingival margin at a 90-degree angle.
- Reinforced Acrylic Pontics (RAPs) is used only for an anterior teeth and maxillary first premolars.
- Advantages of RAPs:
  1. Excellent strength and esthetics.
  2. Usable in a restricted space.
  3. Can be designed so that occlusion is confined to the plastic.
- An indirect retainer should be placed as far from the distal extension base as possible in a prepared rest seat on a tooth capable of supporting its function.
- The use of rugae support for indirect retainer is usually part of a palatal horseshoe design.
- The primary purpose of denture base is to support teeth and effects the transfer of occlusal forces to supporting oral structure.
- The snow shoe principle states that broad coverage of oral structures furnishes the best support with least load per unit area.
- Primary retention for removable partial denture is accomplished by placing retaining elements like clasp on the abutment tooth.
- Stress breakers effectively dissipate vertical stresses.
- Location of the undercut is the most important single factor in selecting a clasp.
- Guiding plane is defined as two or more parallel, vertical surface of abutment teeth, so shaped to direct prosthesis during placement and removal.

Clasping configuration	*Indication*
1. Bilateral configuration	Class I edentulous arch
2. Tripod configuration	Class II edentulous arch
3. Quadrilateral configuration	Class III edentulous arch

- Quadrilateral configuration of clasping is the most effective way to control stress.
- Wrought alloy wire of combination clasp can flex in any spatial plane, whereas a cast clasp flexes in the horizontal plane only. ***(PGI '06)***
- Steps of partial denture design:
  1. 1st step : Determination of support of the partial denture.
  2. 2nd step : Connection of the tooth and tissue support units.
  3. 3rd step : Determination of retention of partial denture.
  4. 4th step : Connection of retention units to the support units.
  5. 5th step : Outline and joining of edentulous area to the already established design components.
- Changes in bone mineralization upto 25% often cannot be recognized by ordinary roentgenographic means.
- Minimum yield strength of 60,000 psi is required for the retentive element of a direct retainer.
- The success or failure of a removable partial denture depends on how well the mouth preparations were accomplished.
- The hydrocolloids impression materials are disinfected with a spray solutions of 2% acid glutaraldehyde, stored in 100% humidity and poured within 1 hour.

- The distal extension removable partial denture depend on the residual alveolar ridge for support, stability and retention. Indirect retainer is also incorporated in it.
- The ideal thickness for the visible light cured denture base materials is 1.5 mm.
- Obturators are prostheses that are used to close maxillary defects and to reestablish a barrier between the oral cavity and the sinus and/or nasal cavities.
- Type of obturators:
  1. Surgical – Placed at the time of surgery
  2. Interim obturator – Placed during the initial post surgical healing period
  3. Definitive obturator – Serves as a long term prostheses after healing.
- The primary indication for placement of a surgical obturator is to immediately reestablish the continuity of the oral cavity.
- Dr. M.M. House classified patients into:
  1. The philosophical.
  2. The exacting.
  3. The hysterical.
  4. The indifferent patient.
- The philosophical patients are the easiest and co-operative to work.
- Torus palatinus occurs twice as often in women as in men and is observed in approximately 20% to 25% of the adult population.
- Torus mandibularis occurs equally in both the sexes and is observed in approximately 5% to 10% of the adult population.

- Partial or total absence of the lamina dura is found in hyperparathyroidism and Paget's disease.
- Akerly classified traumatic vertical overlap into:
  a. Type I : Mandibular incisors extrude and impinge into the palate.
  b. Type II : Mandibular incisors extrude and impinge into the gingival **sulci** of the maxillary incisors.
  c. Type III : Both maxillary and mandibular incisors incline lingually with impingement of the gingival tissues of each arch.
  d. Type IV : Mandibular incisors extrude into the abraded lingual surfaces of the maxillary anterior teeth.
- Kratochvil introduced I-bar removable partial denture.
- **Krol** introduced the RPI system of bar clasp design.
- RPA clasp (rest, proximal plate and Akers clasp) is used in tipped abutments and tissue impingement.
- Examples of Extracoronal attachment are: ASC 52, **Dalbo**, Ceka and Era.
- Example of intracoronal attachment are:
- Stern, Ney and Stern-McCollum.
- Examples of stud attachments: **Dolla** Bona, Rotherman and Gerber.
- Chrome alloy is the material of choice for the metallic framework of a swing-lock removable partile denture.
- Dr. Joe J. Simmons first introduced swing-lock removable partial denture.
- **A.H. Schmidt** first gave the basic principles of removable partial denture design.

- An ideal abutment teeth for clasp design should have 0.010 inch of undercut at the most desired location, either the distobuccal or mesiobuccal line angle and in the gingival third of the clinical crown of the tooth.
- Ney surveyors and Jelenko surveyors differ in that the jelenko arm swivels, whereas the Ney arm is fixed.
- An undercut of 0.020 inch is required if a wrought wire combination clasp is to be used.
- The primary purpose of surveying is to identity the modifications of oral structures that are necessary to fabricate a removable partial denture that will have a successful prognosis.

ADDITIONAL HIGH YIELD FACTS

- **Tripoding** is the method used to have reproducible position of the cast on surveyor.
- Outline of occlusal rest seat is triangular whereas outline of lingual rest seat is slightly rounded 'V' with the apex of 'V' directed incisally and floor of rest seat towards cingulum.
- Nonretentive and stabilizing clasp arms are best located between the middle third and gingival third of the crown rather than on the occlusal third.
- Dental surveyor was first introduced by AJ Fourtunati.

Direct	*Introduced by*
1. Combination clasp	OC Applegate
2. Bar clasp	Ewing Roach
3. Cast circumferential clasp design	Nesbitt
4. Extracoronal attachment (clasp direct retainer)	Henry R Boos
5. Retentive clasp assemblies	WG Bonwill

- Functions of the guiding plane surfaces are:
  1. Provide one path of placement and removal of the restoration.
  2. Ensure the intended actions of reciprocal, stabilizing and retentive components.
  3. Eliminate gross food traps between abutment teeth and components of the denture.
- Main advantage of R.P.D. over fixed partial denture in replacing bilateral lost teeth is cross arch stabilization.
- The major concern of R.P.D. associated with a diabetic patient is unfavourable response of supporting tissue.
- The most rigid palatal major connector is anterior posterior connector.
- The palatal major connector that provides greatest retention is palatal plate.
- The first step in major connector construction is outline of basal seat areas or primary bearing areas.
- The first step in surveying the casts for R.P.D. is establishment of guiding planes. ***(AIPG '06)***
- An indirect retainer in R.P.D. acts to transmits occlusal forces to the teeth other than abutment.
- Relining of the distal extension base is indicated when occlusal contact is lost with rotation about the fulcrum line (or denture).
- The abutment which supports pontics both mesially and distally is called as Pier abutment.
- The main advantage of implant supported prosthesis is maintenance of alveolar bone height.
- Tripod markings are placed on the cast during surveying to record the orientation of the cast to the surveyor.

- Failure of partial dentures due to poor clasp design is best avoided by **altering tooth contours.** *(BHU '06)*
- The mostly used bar clasp assembly is mesio-occlusal rest with the minor connector placed into the **mesiolingual** embrasure, but not contacting the adjacent tooth. *(AIIMS '98)*
- **Heel**-raising movement of a RPD is prevented by indirect retainer.
- Discoloration of a denture constructed from cold cure acrylic resin is due to leaching out of tertiary amines. *(AIPG '94)*
- Looseness seen in a recently delivered RPD is due to deflective occlusal balancing. *(AIIMS '99)*
- Physiologic or functional impression of partial edentulous ridges are:
  1. MC Lean's and Hindel's methods.
  2. Functional relining method.
  3. Fluid wax method.

CHAPTER EIGHT

Fixed Partial Denture

- Three-quarter crowns restore the occlusal surface and three of the four axial surfaces excluding the facial surface.
- Seven-eighths crowns are extensions of the three quarter crown to include a major portion of the facial surface.
- **Pinledge** is an intracoronal restoration which is a modification of an anterior three-quarter crown preparation to obtain primary retention and resistance form long parallel pins.
- The replacement tooth in fixed partial denture is called **pontic**. The teeth that support the FPD are the **abutments.** The restorations that are cemented to the abutments are the retainers. Connector joined retainers to the pontic.
- Diagnostic impressions are commonly made with irreversible hydrocolloid (alginate).
- The alginate impression tray is removed with a quick snap to prevent permanent deformation. ***(BHU '06)***
- Mandibular impression is made with the dentist positioned at the 8 O'clock position and the patient seated at a 45° angle to the floor.

- The maxillary impression is made with the patient in an upright position and the dentist at the **11 O'clock position**.
- For complete mouth radiograph, 14 periapical and 4 bitewing radiographs are essential.
- A pulpless tooth or endodontically treated tooth is contraindicated as an abutment to cantilever fixed partial denture.
- Ante's law states that 'the abutment teeth should have combined pericemental area equal to or greater in pericemental area than the tooth or teeth to be replaced.
- When there is migration (bodily movement) of abutment teeth decreasing mesiodistal length of edentulous area, it requires less pericemental support so the number of abutments used is decreased
- When there is arch form situations creating greater leverage factors the number of abutment in FPD is increased.
- The number of abutments used in FPD is increased for support when mesial or distal tipping or changes in axial inclination of tooth/teeth is present.
- Maxilla.

Type of tooth	*Average root surface area (mm2)*
Central incisor	204
Lateral incisor	179
Caonine	273
First premolar	234
2nd premolar	220
1st molar	433
2nd molar	431

- Mandible

Type of tooth	*Average root surface area (mm2)*
Central incisor	154
Latral incisor	168
Lanine	268
1st premolar	180
2nd premolar	207
1st molar	431
2nd molar	426

- An FPD that occludes with a removable prosthesis is subjected to reduced occlusal loading.
- The mesial one-half crown preparation, the non rigid attachment (semiprecision or stress breakers attachment) and the telescopic prosthesis are recommended for the mesially tilted molar.
- **Odontomyces viscoses** is responsible for cemental caries in the patient **past age 50 years.**
- Caries is always active in the dentiono-enamel junction although the entire carious lesion appears arrested.
- Peeso introduced telescope crowns. It consists of covering the prepared teeth with thin gold copings, that incorporated shoulders at the gingival margin to which a superstructure is abutted with temporary luting agents.
- The three fundamental factors of margin development are definition, uniformity and continuity.
- Indications of laminates are:
  1. Stained/defective restorations.
  2. Diastema.
  3. Fractures.
  4. Attrition.
  5. Adolescent teeth (large pulps).
  6. Discoloration.

- The wrap around of Maryland bridge is 180°. It enhances resistance to lingual displacement, increase the surface area of enamel bonding, and permits bonding to diversely directed enamel rods. ***(BHU '06)***
- **Gingival retraction cord** is kept in the gingival sulcus for 5 to 10 minutes. ***(BHU '06)***
- Among clastomeric impression materials, tear resistance is highest in polysulfide. Shelf life is longest in polyether and elastic recovery is highest in addition silicone (polyvinylsiloxane).

• *Type of temporary crown*	*Indications*
Aluminium shell crown	Premolar and Molars
Preformed metal crowns	Posterior teeth
Preformed polycarbonate crown	Anterior teeth ***(BHU '06)***

- The polycarbonate crown form remains on the tooth preparation, as an integral component for the provisional restoration, whereas the cellulose crown form is removed before cementation of the temporary restoration.
- Three popular resins used to fill the cellulose acetate crown:
  1. Polymethyl methacrylate (most commonly used).
  2. Vinyl polyethyl methacrylate.
  3. Epimine resin.
- TMJ Articulators was introduced by Kenneth Swanson.
- Cement of choice for post and core cementation is glass ionomer cement.
- The overdenture is a complete or removable partial denture fabricated over retained teeth. It is also called **tooth-supported denture, overlay denture, telescope denture** or **hybrid prosthesis.**

• *Type of finish line*	*Indication*
1. Shoulder	Complete porcelain crown, injectable porcelain such as Dicor and Cerestore
2. Beveled shoulder	Porcelain fused to metal (PFM)
3. Chamfer	Posterior crown, lingual surface of anterior ceramic and metal crowns
4. Knife-edge	Pinledge—three quarter crown, younger patients, finish lines on cementum inaccessible areas of the oral cavity

• *Types of pontic*	*Use*
1. Spheroidal pontic	Design of choice in mandibular posterior
2. Modified ridge lap	In maxillary anterior and posterior

- In the **mandibular anterior**, the modified ridge lap is the design of choice when minimal bone loss and esthetics are involved.
- When there is extensive bone loss, elimination of embrasures between pontics is done.
- Ferrule is extension of the axial wall of the crown apical to the missing tooth structure and help in binding the remaining tooth structure together, preventing root fracture of the endodontically treated tooth during function.
- Root canal configurations of maxillary central incisor maxillary first premolar (two roots) mandibular second premolar distobuccal roots of maxillary molars are **circular**.
- Root canal configuration of palatal roots of maxillary molars is **elliptical** in **mesiodistal** direction while the remaining teeth have root canal configuration of elliptical shape in buccolingual direction.

- Whenever possible, the margin of the tooth preparation should be supragingival.
- The most suitable instrument for making a chamfer margin is the tapered diamond with a round tip.
- **Jorgensen** first demonstrated the relationship between the degree of axial wall taper and the magnitude of retention.
- For a crown to seat and have the optimal retention, all axial walls should have a 6-degree from cervical to occlusal.
- Adhesive resin cements are the most retentive of all the type of luting agent.
- Rounding of axial angles and increased taper tend to reduce resistance.
- Rounding the internal line angles reduce stress concentrations and thus increase the retention of the restoration.
- U-shaped grooves or flared boxes provide more resistance than V-shaped ones because the former have walls that are perpendicular to the direction of the applied force.
- **Pontic design classification:**

A Mucosal contact	*B Non-mucosal contact*
1. Ridge lap	1. Sanitary (hygienic)
2. Modified ridge lap	2. Modified sanitary
3. Ovate	
4. Conical (egg. bullet shaped)	

- The saddle or ridge lap pontic has a concave fitting surface that overlaps the residual buccolingually. It is the least hygienic pontic design. ***(BHU '06)***

- The tissue contact of the modified ridge lap should resemble a letter T whose vertical arm ends at the crest of the ridge.
- The ovate pontic is the most esthetically acceptable and ideal form of pontic design.
- Glazed pocelain is considered the most biocompatible of all the pontic materials.
- To lessen occlusal forces and thus the loading of abutment teeth, the buccolingual width of the pontic is reduced by 30%.
- Non rigid connectors are indicated when it is not possible to prepare two abutments for an FPD with a common path of placement.
- Rigid connectors:
  1. Cast connectors.
  2. Soldered connectors.
  3. Soldering gap width.
  4. Loop connectors.
- In soldering gap width rigid connector, an even soldering gap about 0.25 mm is recommended.
- **Loop connectors** are used when an existing diastema is to be maintained in a planned fixed prosthesis. ***(BHU '06)***
- The non rigid connector consists of **mortise** (female component) prepared within the contours of the retainer and a **tenon** (male) attached to the pontic. Mortise and tenon are incorporated in the wax pattern stage.
- Nickel chromium shells are the type of temporary crown used primarily for children with extensively damaged primary teeth.

- A custom tray improves the accuracy of an elastomeric impression by limiting the volume of the material, thus reducing stresses during removal and thermal contraction. ***(BHU '06)***
- The pinledge is indicated for undamaged anterior teeth in dentitions with a low caries incidence while it is contraindicated on nonvital teeth and when the alignment of the abutment will conflict with the proposed path of withdrawal of the fixed partial denture.
- The degree of parallelism between the various aspects of the preparation is the most important single factor in retainer design.
- The loop used in loop connector can be shaped from platinum–gold–palladium alloy wire.

ADDITIONAL HIGH YIELD FACTS

1. Extra retention in abutment teeth is obtained with slots, pins and grooves. ***(AIMS '95)***
2. Wrench like grip is obtained with three fourth crown. ***(AIPG '94)***
3. Partial veneer crown is contraindicated in short teeth. ***(AIIMS '2000)***
4. Repeated fracture of a porcelain fused to metal restoration is primarily due to inadequately designed framework. ***(AIIMS '03)***
5. The effectiveness of condensing porcelain powder to reduce shrinkage is determined by shape and size of the partial. ***(AIIMS '96)***

- Pontic should be convex mesiodistally. ***(AIPG 2000)***
- In fixed partial denture it is better for posterior pontic to avoid balancing side contacts. ***(AIIMS 2k)***

- Flux is used during casting to remove the oxides formed on the gold alloy. ***(AIIMS '94)***
- The length of dowel must be equal to crown length or 2/3rd the length of the root. ***(AIPG '94)***
- The ferrule effect reinforces against vertical root fractures.
- Two primary types of resin bonded bridges with metal retainer are:
  1. Rochette; and
  2. Maryland.
- Rochette type uses small countersunk perforations in the retainer sections for retention and is best suited for anterior bridges. The perforation should be 1.5 to 2 mm apart and have a maximum diameter of 1.5 mm on the tooth side. Each hole is countersunk so that the widest diameter is toward the outside of the retainer.
- Retention in Rochette type is provided by mechanical locking of bonding medium to miroscopic undercuts in the etched enamel and the countersunk holes in the retainer.
- Retention in Maryland bridge is provided by bonding of self-cured resin bonding medium into the microscopic undercuts of both the electrolytially or chemically etched retainer and the etched enamel.
- Adhesion bridges are type of Maryland bridges in which silicoating or a 4-Methacryloxyethyl trimeliate anhydride (4-META) or phosphate ester containing, resin bonding medium is used as a bonding material. These resins are capable of strongly bonding to metal surfaces. Here no electrolytic etching of the surface and chemically bonded to the tooth is done.

CHAPTER NINE

Periodontics

NORMAL PERIODONTIUM AND PERIODONTAL DISEASES

- Histologic depth of normal gingival sulcus is 1.8 mm.
- Probing depth of normal gingival sulcus is 2 to 3 mm.
- The width of the attached gingiva increases with age. ***(PGI '06)***
- **Keratinocyte** is the principal cell type of the gingival epithelium.
- The degree of gingival keratinization diminishes with age and the onset of menopause.
- The length of the normal junctional epithelium ranges from 0.25 to 1.35 mm.
- The junctional epithelium is attached to the tooth surface by means of an internal basal lamina and to the gingival connective tissue by an external basal lamina.
- Keratins K1, K2 , K10, K11 , K12, are specific of epidermal type differentiation.
- K6 and K16 are specific of highly proliferative epithelia.
- K5 and K14 are stratification-specific cytokeratins.

- Gingival fibres consist of type 1 collagen.
- Color of attached and marginal gingiva is produced by vascular supply the thickness and degree of keratinization of the epithelium and the presence of pigment-containing cells.
- Stippling is produced by alternate rounded protuberances and depressions in the gingival surface. The papillary layer of the connective projects into the elevations and the elevated and depressed areas are covered by stratified squamous epithelium.
- Principal fibers are composed of collagen type I, reticular fibers are composed of collagen type III and basal lamina is composed of collagen type IV.
- The periodontal ligament is narrowest in the region of the axis of rotation and is shaped like an hourglass.
- The permeability of cementum decreases with age.
- Cementum is thicker in distal surfaces than in mesial surfaces of the root.
- Hypercementosis of the entire dentition occur in patients with Paget's disease.
- Bone contains 99% of calcium ions of the body.
- The organic matrix of bone consists of 90% of collagen type I.
- Neisseria gonorrhoeae and Treponema pallidum increases the prevalence of gingival disease.
- Candida albicans causes gingival diseases in immunocompromised patients.
- Herpes viruses causes gingival diseases.
- Periodontitis is observed in the following systemic diseases:

a. Papillon-Lefevre syndrome by down syndrome.
b. Down syndrome.
c. Leukocyte adhesion deficiency syndromes.
d. Neutropenia (acquired and familial).
e. Chediak Higashi syndrome.
f. Cohen syndrome.
g. Glycogen storage disease.
h. Hypophosphatasia.
i. Leukaemia.
j. Histiocytosis syndromes.

Mnemonic: **PDL N**ational **C**adet **C**orps, **G**rowth, **H**ormone, **L**utenizing **H**ormone

- The initial bacteria colonizing the pellicle-coated tooth surface are predominantly gram positive facultative micro-organisms such as Actinomyces viscosus and streptococcus sangins.
- Non-specific plaque hypothesis was given by Walter Loesche.
- The hallmark of periodontitis is the loss of connective tissue attachment to the tooth.
- Collagenase is produced by P. gingivalis and A. actino-mycetemcomitans.
- **Gingipains** are a group of related proteases produced by Porphyromonas gingivalis.
- Ehler Danlos syndrome (Type IV, VIII, IX) has a defect in Type III collagen.
- Papillon-Levre syndrome has a defect in Cathepsin C (dipeptidyl aminopeptidase I).
- Hypophosphatasia has a defect in alkaline phosphatase enzyme. So alkaline phosphatase cannot function normally.

- The crystal forms of inorganic component of calculus are: **H**ydroxyapatite, **m**agnesium whitlockite, **o**ctacalcium phosphate, **b**rushite
  Mnemonic: My **HBO** channel
- Saliva is the source of mineralization for supragingival calculus while gingival crevicular fluid is the source of mineralization for subgingival calculus.
- Calcification begins along the inner surface of the supragingival plague and in the attached component of subgingival plaque adjacent to the tooth.
- Saliva production is permanently impaired when salivary glands receive ≥ 6000 rad (1cGY = 1 nad). *(AIPG '05)*
- In aleukemic leukemia, patients have normal blood counts while leukaemic cells are present in the bone marrow.
- **In leukemia cutis**, there is abnormal accumulation of leukemic cells in the dermal and subcutaneous connective tissue and forms elevated flat macules and papules.
- Periotron is an electronic transducer used to measure the amount of gingival crevicular fluid (GCF).
- Saliva contains coagulation factor VIII, IX, X, XI, XII.
- Perivascular precipitation of metallic sulfides in the subepithelial connective tissue results in gingival pigmentation.
- Diseases that increase melanin pigmentation are:
  i. **A**ddison's diseases.
  ii. **P**eutz-Jeghers syndrome.
  iii. **A**lbright's syndrome.

iv. Von Recklinghausen's disease (**n**eurofibromatosis).
Mnemonic: PAAN

- Cyclosporine induced gingival enlargement is more frequent in children.

Drugs	*% of occurrence of gingival enlargement*
Phenytoin	50% of patients taking the drug
Cyclosporine	30% of patients taking the drugs
Nifedipine	20% of patients taking the drugs

- Bacterial plague is necessary for the initiation of conditioned enlargement i.e. in pregnancy, puberty, vitamin C deficiency, plasma cell gingivitis.
- Angiogranuloma is gingival enlargement in pregnancy. ***(PGI '06)***
- Gingival enlargement in vitamin C deficiency is marginal.
- Capnocytophaga sp. is involved in pubertal gingivitis.
- Leukemic gingival enlargement is due to leukocytic infiltration. ***(PGI '06)***
- **Squamous cell carcinoma** is the most common malignant tumor of the gingiva.
- Primary herpetic gingivostomatitis occurs most often in infants and children younger than 6 years of age.
- **Chronic marginal gingivitis** is the most prevalent type of gingival change in childhood.
- Immunofluorescent technique can detect the presence of autoantibodies in the oral mucosa of oral pemphigus patients.
- In surprabony pocket, the pattern of destruction of the underlying bone is horizontal while in intrabony pocket the done destructive pattern is vertical.

- Horizontal bone loss is the most common pattern of bone loss in periodontal diseases.
- The most clinical sign of trauma to the periodontium is increased tooth mobility. ***(AIIMS '06)***
- Chaput gave the term 'Juvenile periodontitis'.
- Vertical loss of alveolar bone around the first molars and incisors, beginning around puberty in otherwise healthy teenagers, is a classic diagnostic sign of localized aggressive periodontitis.
- Candidiasis is the most common oral lesion in HIV diseases and has been found in approximately 90% of AIDS patients.

DIAGNOSIS AND TREATMENT OF PERIODONTAL DISEASE

- The long cone paralleling technique projects the most realistic image of the level of the alveolar bone.
- Bone loss is always greater than it appears in the radiograph.
- In scleroderma, the periodontal ligament is uniformly widened at the expense of the surrounding alveolar bone.
- Bleeding on probing is the best clinical indicator of gingival inflammation.
- Prognosis is established after the diagnosis is made and before the treatment plan is established.
- More closer the center of rotation of tooth to the crown, more favourable is the distribution of occlusal forces to the periodontium and hence the prognosis.
- The Perio Temp probe measure the temperature in the gingival tissue.

- **The Foster-Miller probe** described by Jeffcoat *et al.* detects cemento-enamel junction and pocket depth. ***(AIPG '06)***
- **Florida probe** measures relative clinical attachment levels.
- Subtraction radiography facilitates both qualitative and quantitative visualization of even minor density changes in bone by removing the unchanged anatomic structure from the image.
- **Darkfield or phase contrast microscopy** has been suggested as an alternative to culture methods on the basis of its ability to directly and rapidly assess the morphology and motility of bacteria in a plague sample. ***(AIPG '06)***
- **Fujise** ***et al.*** developed a Polymerase Chain Reaction assays that have the potential for being an ideal detection method of periodontal microorganisms.
- Regeneration of the periodontium is a continuous physiologic process.
- The amount of drug excreted in breast milk is not more than 1% to 2% of the maternal dose.
- Scaling and root planning is safe unless platelet counts are < 60,000/mm^3.
- Surgical procedures is indicated when the platelet count is > 80,000/mm^3.
- **D**iuretics, **a**ntihistamines **t**ricyclic antidepressants and **a**ntihypertensives cause xerostomia. (mnemonic: DATA).
- Radiation treatment for oral, head, neck, and thyroid cancers, Sjögren's syndrome; poorly controlled diabetes; bone marrow transplantation thyroid disorders and depression are associated with dry mouth.

- Curettes are the best instruments for subgingival scaling and root planning because they provide the best adaptation to complex root anatomy.
- **Gracey curettes** and their area of use:
  Gracey # 1-2 and 3-4: Anterior teeth
  Gracey # 5-6 : Anterior teeth and premolars
  Gracey # 7-8 and 9-10: posterior teeth : facial and lingual
  Gracey # 11-12 : posterior teeth: mesial
  Gracey # 13-14 : posterior teeth: distal
- Offset blade of the Gracey curettes are angled approximately 60 to 70 degrees from the lower shank.
- Tip action of sonic scaler is orbital.
- Tip action of magnetostrictive ultrasonic scaler is elliptical while that of piezoelectric ultrasonic scaler is linear.
- Prophy-jet delivers an air-powered slurry of warm water and sodium bicarbonate.
- Electrosurgery (radiosurgery) uses controlled high-frequency electrical (radio) currents in the range of 1.5 to 7.5 million cycles per second or megahertz.
- Scaling stroke is short, powerful pull stroke while light pull stroke is used in root planning.
- **Gracey curettes** were designed by Dr. Clayton H. Gracey.
- 3% H_2O_2 is used in treatment of necrotizing ulcerative gingivitis.
- For children, the brush is smaller, thinner (0.005 inch or 0.1 mm) and shorter (0.344 inch or 8.7 mm) bristles as compared to adult. ***(BHU '06)***
- Bristle hardness is proportional to the square of the diameter and inversely proportional to the square of bristle length.

- Circular motion of brushing is used in the Fones technique of brushing.
- Back and forth motion on occlusal surfaces of the teeth is used with the Bass, Stillman and Charters method of brushing.

Brushing method	Indications
1. The Bass method	Any patient with or without periodontal involvement
2. The modified Stillman method	Patient with gingival recession and root exposure
3. The Charters method	Areas of healing wounds after periodontal surgery

- Dental floss is the most effective dental hygiene aid for cleaning in narrow gingival embrasures that are occupied by intact papillae and bordered by tight contact zones.
- Massaging the gingiva with toothbrush or an interdental cleaning devices produces epithelial thickening increased keratinization and increased mitotic activity in the epithelium and connective tissue.

• *Local delivery product*	*Antimicrobial agent*
Actisite	Tetracyline
Atridox	Doxycyline
Elyzol ***(AIPG '06)***	Metronidazole
Periochip	Chlorhexidine

- **Papilla preservation flap** is the technique of choice when osseous defects amenable to regeneration are present.
- Complete epithelial repair after gingivectomy takes place at about 1 month while complete connective tissue repair takes about 7 weeks.

- The flow of gingival fluid is initially increased after gingivectomy and diminishes as healing progresses. Maximal flow is reached after 1 week.
- Healing after flap surgery: One week after surgery: epithelial attachment to the root by means of hemi-desmosomes and a basal lamina.
  Two weeks after surgery: Collagen fibres begin to appear parallel to the tooth surface.
  One month after surgery: A fully epithlialized gingival crevice with a well-defined epithelial attachment.
- Ramfjord and Nissle gave the term modified Widman flap.
- Indications of gingivectomy technique:
  1. Elimination of suprabony pockets if the pocket wall is fibrous and firm.
  2. Elimination of gingival enlargement.
  3. Elimination of suprabony periodontal abscesses.
- The flap technique for pocket therapy are:
  1 The Modified Widman flap.
  2. The Undisplaced palatal flap.
  3. The apically displaced flap.
- Flaps for regenerative surgery are:
  1. The papilla preservation flap.
  2. Conventional flap.
- **Transgingival probing** or sounding detects the extent and configuration of the intrabony component of the pocket or furcation defects. ***(PGI '06)***
- Osseous resective surgery is done for treatment of interproximal craters exostoses, one wall angular defect.
- The flap technique best suited for grafting purposes is the papilla preservation flap because it provides

complete coverage of the interdental area after suturing.

- Examples of Autogenous bone grafts are Osseous coagulum intraoral cancellons bone marrow transplants, bone swaging, iliac autografts.
- Undecalcified freeze-dried bone, decalcified freeze dried bone are allografts.
- Calf bone, Kiel bone, Anorganic bone are xenografts.
- Sclera, cartilage, plaster of paris, calcium phosphate biomaterials like hydroxyapatite and tricalcium phosphate, plastic materials like HTR polymer, bioactive glass coral derived materials are non bone graft materials.
- The primary etiologic factor in the development of furcation defects is bacterial plague and the inflammatory consequences that result from its long-term presence.
- Techniques used for gingival augmentation coronal to the recession (root coverage) are:
  1. Free gingival autograft.
  2. Free connective tissue autograft.
  3. Pedicle autografts:
     - Laterally (horizontally) positioned.
     - Coronally positioned.
     - Semilunar pedicle.
  4. Subepithelial connective tissue graft.
  5. Guided tissue regeneration.
  6. Pouch and tunnel technique.
- Sullivan and Atkins classified gingival recessions into four morphologic categories:
  1. Shallow – narrow
  2. Shallow – wide

3. Deep – narrow
4. Deep – wide

- **Free Gingival Autograft** was described by Miller.
- Free connective tissue autograft was described by Levin.
- Laterally (horizontally) displaced pedicle autograft was described by Grupe and Warren.
- In Pouch and Tunnel technique of root coverage, the subepithelial donor connective tissue is placed into pouches beneath papillary tunnels. This allows for intimate contact of donor tissue to the recipient site. It minimize incisions and reflection of flaps and provide abundant blood supply to the donor tissue.
- **Branemark** used implants for the first time.
- An important difference between periimplant and periodontal tissues is that collagen fibres are non attached and run parallel to the implant surface, owing to the lack of cementum.
- In the two-stage implant surgical approach, the implants are left undisturbed for 2 to 3 months in the mandible whereas in the maxilla 4 to 6 months because of slower healing due to less dense bone.
- In drilling hole for implant placement in the bone, the drill is used at a speed of 800 to 1000 rpm with copious irrigation to prevent overheating the bone.

Non-resorbable barrier membranes	*Resorbable barrier membranes*
1. Latex	1. Polyglycolic acid
2. Teflon (e- PTFE, Gore Tex, Flagstaff, AZ)	2. Polylacitic acid
	3. Trimethylene carbonate

Biologic properties of various bone graft materials

	Osteconductive	*Osteoinductive*	*Steoginic*
Autograft	Yes	Yes	Yes
Autograft	Yes	Yes/No	No
Xenograft	Yes	No	No
Alloplast	Yes	No	No

- An implant-assisted denture is designed so that most of the masticatory load is borne by the primary denture support (stress bearing) areas like retromolar pad buccal shelf.

ADDITIONAL HIGH YIELD FACTS

- Stippling is absent in both infants and old people. *(AIPG '97)*
- Occlusal forces are tolerated mostly by oblique fibers of periodontal ligament. *(AIIMS 2000)*
- Principal fibers of the periodontal ligament are collagenous fibers. *(AIPG '03)*
- Junctional epithelium is very susceptible to infection because it has a high turnover rate of cells. *(AIPG '96)*
- Gingiva in children is more keratinised but less stippled as compared to that of adult.
- Predominant bacteria found in two days old plaque is streptococci. *(AIPG '98, BHU '06)*
- Amount of water in plague is 80%. *(PGI '98)*
- The predominant cell type in gingival crevicular fluid is polymorphonuclear leukocyte. *(AIPG '03)*
- IgG immuonglobulin is present in high concentration in gingival crevicular fluid. *(AIIMS May '06)*

- A. actinomycetemcomitans produce leukotoxin which has toxic affect on neutrophils.
- Gingival recession is most commonly caused by tooth brush trauma. ***(AIIMS '95)***
- The gingival enlargement in leukaemia mainly results from leukemic cellular infiltration of gingiva. ***(PGI June '06)***
- Gingival enlargement in pregnancy is termed as angiogranuloma. ***(PGI June '06)***
- Pyogenic granuloma is a mass of granulation tissue with chronic inflammatory cellular infiltration. Treatment consists of removal of the lesions plus the elimination of irritating local factors. The recurrence rate is about 15%.
- Pregnancy associated gingivitis is accompanied by increases in steroid hormones in crevicular fluid and increases in the levels of Prevotella intermedia, which uses the steroids as growth factors.
- The connective tissue wall of a periodontal pocket is densely infiltrated with plasma cells (approximately 80%). ***(AIIMS '92)***
- "Mirror image" type of bone loss pattern is seen in localized juvenile periodontits.
- In Papillon-Lefevre syndrome, there is untimely loss of primary and permanent teeth due to severe destruction of periodontium.
- Standard force for evaluating periodontal pockets that is well toterated is 0.75 N or 25 g. ***(AIPG '95)***
- Kirkland and Orban knives are used for gingivectomy.
- Effective use of dental floss can be expected to improve gingival health. ***(AIPG '04)***

- First group of fibres damaged in periodontitis is dentogingival fibers.
- The oxygen consumption of normal gingival is 1.6 ± 0.37. *(AIPG '05)*
- Hypercementosis with hyperplasia at root apex is associated with hypo function. *(AIPG '94)*
- If content of ammonia is increased in saliva it results in decrease in plague formation. *(AIPG '97)*
- Most aggressive bacteria penetrating connective tissue and resulting in bone destruction is present in **sub-gingival epithelial attached plague**.
- Clinical signs of gingivitis first appear in early or Stage II gingivitis.
- McCall festoons is life preserver shaped enlargement of marginal gingiva and are common in canine and premolar area.
- Down's syndrome is characterized by low prevalence of caries but high prevalence of periodontitis.
- Diseases presenting clinically as desquamative gingivitis are:
  1. **L**ichen planus
  2. **P**emphigoid
     - Bullous pemphigoid
     - Cicatrial pemphigoid
  3. **P**emphigus vulgaris
  4. **C**hronic ulcerative stomatitis
  5. **L**inear Ig A dermatosis
  6. **Lu**pus erythematosis
  7. Erythema multiforme
  8. **D**ermatitis herpetiformis

  Mnemonic: LDC LUMP LiP

- Mouth mirror used by dentist is a concave mirror.

Type of suture	*Indication*
1. Horizontal mattress suture	Interproximal areas of diastemata or for wide interdental spaces for adaptation of interproximal papilla against the bone
2. Continuous independent sling	Adaptation of facial and lingual flap suture involving many teeth
3. Anchor suture	Closing of flap mesial or distal to a tooth
4. Periosteal suture	Holding place apically displaced partial thickness flap

- Gore Tex membrane is used during reattachment procedures to prevent formation of long junctional epithelium. ***(BHU '06)***
- Histologically phenytoin induced hyperplasia depicts proliferation of fibroblast-like cells and epithelium.
- The process of keratinisation is closely associated with acid phosphatase enzyme.
- The antibody which is most resistant to proteolysis is secretory IgA.

CHAPTER TEN

Community Dentistry

(Including Preventive and Social Medicine)

- Father of Epidemmology is John Snow.
- Components of Epidemiology are:
  1. Disease frequency.
  2. Distribution of disease.
  3. Determinants of disease.
- Epidemiological triad consist of the agent, the host and the environment.
- In a proportion, the numerator is always a part of the denominator.
- Secondary attack rate is defined as "the number of persons exposed to the risk factor developing the disease within the range of the incubation period following exposure to a primary case".
- Prevalence = Incidence × Mean duration.
- **Bimodality** is the occurrence of separate peaks in an age-incidence of a disease for e.g. Hodgkin's disease.
- Odds ratio is used for calculation of the association of an exposure and a disease in a case control study.

Association between smoking of cigarettes and development of leukoplakia

Risk factor (Smoking)	*Cases*	*Controls*
Present	a	b
Absent	c	d

$$\text{Odds ratio} = \frac{a \times d}{b \times c}$$

- Theories of caries formation:
  1. Acidogenic theory by Miller.
  2. Proteloysis theory by Gottleib.
  3. Proteolysis chelation theory by Schatz and Martin.
- The pH of saliva is determined mainly by the concentration of bicarbonate.
- Sialin is an arginine peptide and is a pH rise factor.
- Vipeholm study by Gustafsson *et al.* showed that the physical form of carbohydrates is much more important in causing caries than the total amount of sugar ingested.
- Bis-biguanides like chlorhexidine and alexidine have both hydrophobic and hydrophilic constituents and possessing a net positive charge at physiologic pH.
- Caries vaccine helps in controlling caries by interfering with bacterial growth and metabolism.
- Caries risk, regardless of the age of the patient, is a major criterion for selecting teeth for sealant application.
- Caries activity tests:
  1. **Lactobacillus colony count test:**
     Hadley introduced it and is related to caries susceptibility of a person.

2. **Snyder test:**
   It measures the ability of salivary micro-organisms to form organic acids from carbohydrate.
3. **The Swab test:**
   Grainger developed it and is used in evaluating caries activity in very young children.
4. **Alban test:**
   It is simplified version for Snyder test.

FLUORIDES

- Fluorides control caries activity by altering the tooth surface or contour.
- The intake of fluoride by tea drinkers is in the range of 0.04 to 2.7mg/day.
- Fluoride concentration of human milk ranges from 6-12 mg/ml.
- The maximum plasma concentration of fluoride following the oral intake of fluoride on a fasting stomach is reached within 30 minutes and this is independent of the amount of fluoride ingested.
- The **plasma half life** fluoride is in range of **4-10 hours.**
- 99% of all fluoride in the human body is found in calcified tissues (apatite crystals).
- Absorption of soluble fluoride by gastrointestinal tract and sometimes by lungs is 82-97% of the ingested fluoride.
- Total fluoride content cementum increases with age.
- Fluoride concentration of extracellular fluid and plasma is more than intracellular fluid.
- Fluoride concentration decreases in the order: Plasma > Saliva > Breast milk.

- Reduction of dental caries by community water fluoridation is 50-65%.
- The most common form of systemic fluoride administration is fluoridation—the addition of fluoride to public water supplies.
- Fluoride content in plague is in the range of 15-64 ppm.

Topical fluoride compounds	*Introduced by:*
1. Sodium fluoride	Bibby, Knutson, co-workers
2. Stannous fluoride	Muhler *et al.*
3. Acidulated phosphate	Brudevold *et al.*
4. Amine fluoride	Muhlemann *et al.*

- Comparison of topical fluoride agents:

Characteristic	*NaF*	*SnF_2*	*APF*
1. Percent fluoride	2%	8%	1.23%
2. Ppm fluoride	9200	19,500	12,300
3. Effectiveness	29%	30%	28%

- Stannous fluoride undergoes rapid hydrolysis and oxidation and forms stannous hydroxide and stamina ion. Therefore, a fresh solution is prepared for each treatment.
- Acidulated phosphate fluoride application results in surface roughening of porcelain or composite restorations if it is used repeatedly and for a prolonged time.
- Sodium fluoride application is recommended for public health programs.
- Bibby did the first clinical trial of fluoride dentifrice by using sodium fluoride.
- Premolars are usually affected first by fluorosis and mandibular incisors are last to be affected.

- Plasma level of fluoride at the appearance of dental fluorosis is above 2 µm/litre for chronic ingestion and 10 µm/litre for and acute ingestion.

Toxic effect of excessive chronic ingestion of fluoride

Effect	*Dosage*	*Duration*
1. Dental fluorosis	> 2 ppm	until 5 years
2 Skeletal fluorosis	10-25 mg/day	10-20 years
3. Kidney damage	5-10mg/1kg	6-12 months

- The first community water fluoridation was done in Grand Rapids, USA in 1945. *(AIPG '06)*
- Fluoride compounds used in water fluoridation are:
  1. Fluorspar.
  2. Sodium fluoride-most expensive source.
  3. Silico fluorides.
  4. Sodium silicofluoride.
  5. Ammonium silicofluoride.
  6. Hydrofluosilicic acid.
- Equipments for water fluoridation are:
  1. Saturator system.
  2. Dry-feeder system.
  3. Solution-feeder system.
  4. Venturi fluoridator system.
  5. Saturation suspension.
- **The Nalgonda technique** defluoridation is used to remove excess fluoride from water and keep the water in desirable levels.
- The process of defluoridation of water by Nalgonda technique involves the sequential addition of lime, bleaching powder and filter alum to the fluoride water followed by flocculation, sedimentation and filtration.

- *Composition of dentifrices (tooth paste)*

Component	*Content in %*	*Examples*
1. Abrasive	40-50%	Calcium pyrophosphate, sodium metaphosphate dicalcium phosphate
2. Humectant	20%-50%	Glycerol, sorbitol propylene glycol
3. Binders or thickening agent	0.5-2%	Sodium alginate methyle cellulose, sodium carboxyl methylcellulose
4. Detergent or surfaces active agent	1-2%	Sodium lauryl sulphate sodium-N lauryl sarcosinate sodium alkyle sulfoacetate
5. Flovouring agents, colour	1-4%	
6. Fluoride	0-1%	Sodium monofluorophosphate
7. Water	20-30%	

• *Internal cleaners*	*Type of embrasure*	*Indications*
Dental floss	I	No gingival recession
Interdental brush	II	Moderate papillary recession
Uni-tufted brush	III	Complete loss of interdental papillae

- **Loe and Schiott** first used 0.2% chlorhexidine gluconate of plague control.
- Scrub technique of tooth brushing is the most commonly used technique.
- Schroeder introduced the use of chlorhexidine as antiplague agent.
- Chlorhexidine is prepared with digluconate salt to make it more water soluble.
- First generation antiplague compounds are antibiotics phenols, quaternary ammonium compounds and sanguinarine 20 to 50% reduction of plague scores is achieved.

- Second Generation antiplague compounds are bisbiguanides enzymes etc. 70% to 90% reduction of plague scores is achieved.
- Bowen's disease is a localized, intraepidermal squamous carcinoma.
- Leukoplakia is the most common precancerous lesion.
- The etiology of leukoplakia is six "S"s viz. smoking, spirits, spices, sharp tooth edge sepsis and syphilis.
- The most common site of occurrence of oral submuccous fibrosis is buccal mucosa.
- Mrs. Irene Newman is considered as the first dental hygienist.
- **Dr. Fones** is considered as the father of dental hygiene.
- The Dentist Act was passed on 1948.
- The Indian Dental Association was formed on 1949.
- The World Health Organization was formed on 7th April 1948.
- The Oral Health Unit of WHO was established in 1956.
- The World Health Day theme of 1994 was "Oral Health for a Healthy life".
- Group Health Education Methods:
  1. *Symposiums:* It is useful in delivering health education to a group of adults who have an attitude for listening and the ability to appreciate the topic presented.
  2. *Group discussions:* A group leader starts and conducts the discussion and give every one of the audience to actively participate.
  3. *Buzz sessions (Small group discussion):* It is the most informal form of communication.

4. *Panel discussions:* The audience is allowed to ask questions and clarify their doubts.
5. *Colloquy:* A group of experts along with the active participation of audience discuss specific problems and find solutions.
6. *Workshops:* It is problem solving method and useful for people with previous experience on particular topics and for institutions and departments.

- **Pathfinder survey** is a stratified cluster sampling technique, that includes the most important population subgroups likely to have differing disease levels and to cover all subjects in specific index age group in any one location.
- Index age and age groups for pathfinder survey are 5 years for primary teeth and 12, 15, 35–44 and 65–74 years for permanent teeth.
- Types of pathfinder surveys:
  1. Pilot survey.
  2. National pathfinder survey.
- Functions of the primary health center includes training of health guides, health workers, local dais and health assistants.
- Community health center covers a population of 80000 to 120000.

Indices used to asses oral hygiene and their proponent

	Index	*Proponent*
1.	Oral hygiene index simplified (OHI –S)	Greene & vermillion
2.	Plague Index	Quigley and Hein
3.	Papillary mariginal attached gingival index (PMA)	Massler X Schour
4	Gingival index (GI)	Loe and Silness
5.	Periodontal Index (PI)	Russell
6.	Periodontal Disease Index (PDI)	Ramfjord

- The clinical status of oral hygiene can be known from scores of simplified oral hygiene index. (OHI-S):
  1. Good – 0.0 to 1.2
  2. Fair – 1.3 to 3.0
  3. Poor – 3.1 to 6.0
- Ramfjord teeth are maxillary right first molar, maxillary left central incisor, maxillary left first premolar, mandibular left first molar, mandibular right central incisor and mandibular right first premolar.
- The periodontal index score of 8 indicates advanced destruction of bone with loss masticatory function.
- Decayed-Missing-Filled Index (DMF Index) was introduced by Klein, Palmer, Knutson and it is applied only to permanent teeth.
- The 'def' index was described by Gruebbel and it is applicable to primary teeth.
- Root Caries Index was described by V. Katz.
- Fluorosis Index was given by H. Dean.
- The TNM system for staging of oral cancer was developed by Pierre Denoix.
- The "Community Periodontal Index of Treatment Needs" was developed by Ainamo *et al.*
- The CPITN probe has black mark from 3.5 mm to 5.5 mm.
- The working force of CPITN probe is 25 gms.

BIOSTATISTICS

- **John Graunt** is considered as the father of Health Statistics.
- Discrete quantitative data takes only fixed values like whole numbers while continuous quantitative data takes any value, decimal or fractional.

- **Lottery method** is a type of simple random sampling.
- Line diagram is the simplest type of diagram.
- Measures of central tendency are mean, median and mode.
- Measures of dispersion used in community dentistry are range, standard deviation and coefficient of variation.
- Dispersion is defined as the degree of spread or variation of the variable about a central value.
- Coefficient of variation is given by the formula: $(S \times 100)/\bar{x}$

  where S = standard deviation

  $\bar{x}$ = mean
- The area under normal distribution or the gaussian distribution curve is calculated in terms of a relationship between the mean and standard deviation is as follows:

  a. Mean ± 1 S.D. covers 68.3% of the observations.

  b. Mean ± 2 S.D. covers 95.4% of the observations.

  c. Mean ± 3 S.D. covers 99.7% of the observations.
- Standard errors of proportion is given by:

  $\sqrt{\{(pq)/n\}}$ where

  p = proportion of occurrence of an event in the sample

  q = 1 – p

  n = sample size
- Standard error of mean is given by

  $SD/\sqrt{n}$ where SD = standard devuation

  n = sample size

- Paired t-test is used when an individual gives a pair of observations eg. amount of plague accumulation on tooth after and before chlorhexidine mouthrinses.
- Correlation is the relationship between two sets of variable. The degree of relationship between two variables is known as correlation coefficient. Correlation coefficient range is denoted as $-1 \leq r \leq +1$ where r is correlation coefficient.
- Chi-square test (X^2) uses nominal data and is a test of proportion.

ADDITIONAL HIGH YIELD FACTS

- The indicators of physical quality of life index are infant mortality, life expectancy at age one and literacy.
- The denominator in child mortality rate is child of ages 1-4 years. ***(AIIMS May '06)***
- In primordial prevention, prevention of the emergence or development of risk factor done.
- The basis of mortality data is the Death Certificate.
- The WHO declared that smallpox had been eradicated on 1980.
- Methods of chlorination of water are chlorine gas, chloramines, perchloron.
- The point at which the chlorine demand of the water is met is called the "break-point". Free chlorine like HOCL and OCl begins to appear in water if further chlorine is added beyond the break point.
- Sensitivity $= \frac{\text{Number of subjects who test positive}}{\text{Number of subject with disease}}$

- Specificity $= \dfrac{\text{Number of subjects who test negative}}{\text{Number of subject with disease}}$
- Positive predictive value =

$$\frac{\text{True positive}}{\text{All patients with positive test results (false + true positive)}}$$

- Negative predictive value of the test is the probability that a person with a negative test does not have the disease.

  Negative predictive value =

$$\frac{\text{True negative}}{\text{True negative + false positive}}$$

- Under the National Programme for control of Blindness **school teachers** are supposed to conduct the vision screening of school student.
- Color-coding of bag in hospitals to dispose off human anatomical wastes such as body parts is **yellow**.
- Multipurpose worker scheme in India was introduced following the recommendation of **Kartar Singh Committee.**
- Basic Health Service scheme in India was introduced following the recommendation of Mukherji Committee.
- Most important epidemiological tool used for assessing disability in children is Wing's Handicaps, Behaviour and Skills Schedule.
- The biological oxygen demand indiates organic matter.

- Gap between a primary and a secondary case is **serial interval**.
- Reverse cold chain is used for carrying stool samples of polio patients from a Primary Health Center to the laboratory.
- Most common cause of infant mortality rate in India is low birth weight (prematurity).
- Hospice refers to special group of people helping the old and terminally ill patients.
- Osmolality of WHO Oral Rehydration salt is 300 (WHO Oral Rehydration Salt).
- The national health policy is based on comprehensive health care.
- Sentinel surveillance is done to know the hidden cases in community.
- International certificate for travelling is required for yellow fever.
- **Incidence of diarrhoea** in a community can be calculated by **Cohort Study**.
- Denominator in birth rate is mid year population.
- The major purpose of randomization in a clinical trial is to ensure the groups are comparable on base line characteristics.
- The standard normal distribution has variance = 1.
- The usefulness of a screening test in community depends on its sensitivity.
- The parameters of sensitivity and specificity are used for assessing discriminant validity.
- Sampling error is classified as alpha error.

- Confidence limits includes mean and standard error.
- Two variables can be plotted together in scatter diagram.
- The number of degree of freedom in table of (4 × 4) is 9.
  Degree of freedom = (c–1) × (r–1)
  Where, C =
  R = no. of rows—Therefore,
  (4–1)(4–1) = 9
- When an intervention is applied to community to evaluate its usefulness, it is termed as trial for **effectiveness.**
- When a drugs is evaluated for its usefulness in controlled conditions, it is termed as a trial signifying **efficacy**.
- Low birth weight statistics of a hospital is best shown by histogram.
- The most effective way of health education is setting an example.
- Concept of Primary Health Center (PHC) was devised at Alma Atta in erstwhile USSR.
- Soiling index is an indicator of air pollution.
- Venturi meter is used for measuring bed strength in slow sand filter.
- Histogram is used to describe quantitative data of a group of patient.
- **Horrock's apparatus** is used for the estimation of chlorine demand of water.

- The daily use of fluoride gel in custom trays at home is indicated in the following situations:
  1. Rampant enamel or root caries in any age group.
  2. Xerostomia.
  3. Head and neck radiation therapy.
  4. For use on abutment teeth under an overdenture.
  5. Hypersensitive root surfaces.
- Chi-square test is used to measure the degree of agreement between two observations.
- A measure of location which divides the distribution in the ratio of 3:1 is **third quartile**.
- Immediate treatment of a child who accidentally swallows 10 ml of 10% fluoride solution is to give the child copious amount of milk.
- The first step in public health procedure is survey of problem.
- Defluoridation is an example of primary level of prevention.
- Vaccine for caries is based on Ig A immunoglobulin.
- The foolproof method to check the diet counselling is lactobacillus test.
- Most effective way to control caries at home is acidulated phosphate fluoride gel.
- 2% NaF can be used in ceramic restoration.
- Fluoride is carried in the blood via plasma.
- The fluoride form that has to be freshly prepared before use is stannous fluoride. ***(AIPG '97)***